WATER FITNESS LESSON PLANS

AND

CHOREOGRAPHY

CHRISTINE ALEXANDER

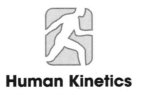

Human Kinetics

Library of Congress Cataloging-in-Publication Data

Alexander, Christine, 1950-
   Water fitness lesson plans and choreography / Christine Alexander.
        p. cm.
   Includes bibliographical references.
   ISBN-13: 978-0-7360-9112-1 (soft cover)
   ISBN-10: 0-7360-9112-2 (soft cover)
   1. Aquatic exercises. I. Title.
   GV838.53.E94A44 2011
   613.7'16--dc22

                                                    2010030738

ISBN-10: 0-7360-9112-2 (print)
ISBN-13: 978-0-7360-9112-1 (print)

Copyright © 2011 by Christine Alexander

The Web addresses cited in this text were current as of July 22, 2010, unless otherwise noted.

Acquisitions Editor: Gayle Kassing, PhD; **Managing Editor:** Amy Stahl; **Assistant Editor:** Rachel Brito; **Copyeditor:** Patsy Fortney; **Permission Manager:** Dalene Reeder; **Graphic Designer:** Bob Reuther; **Graphic Artists:** Kathleen Boudreau-Fuoss and Yvonne Griffith; **Cover Designer:** Keith Blomberg; **Photographer:** James Wiseman; **Visual Production Assistant:** Joyce Brumfield; **Photo Production Manager:** Jason Allen; **Printer:** United Graphics

We thank Oak Point Recreation Center in Plano, Texas, for assistance in providing the location for the photo shoot for this book.

All text from *Going Deep* by Craig Stuart (2009) is printed or placed online with written permission of the publisher, Hanley-Wood, LLC.

Following is contact information for the United States Water Fitness Association from whom text is cited in this book:

United States Water Fitness Association
P.O. Box 243279, Boynton Beach, FL 33424-3279
Telephone: (561) 732-9908, E-mail: info@uswfa.org, Web site: www.uswfa.org

Printed in the United States of America   10 9 8 7 6 5 4 3 2 1

The paper in this book is certified under a sustainable forestry program.

Human Kinetics
Web site: www.HumanKinetics.com

United States: Human Kinetics
P.O. Box 5076
Champaign, IL 61825-5076
800-747-4457
e-mail: humank@hkusa.com

Canada: Human Kinetics
475 Devonshire Road Unit 100
Windsor, ON N8Y 2L5
800-465-7301 (in Canada only)
e-mail: info@hkcanada.com

Europe: Human Kinetics
107 Bradford Road
Stanningley
Leeds LS28 6AT, United Kingdom
+44 (0) 113 255 5665
e-mail: hk@hkeurope.com

Australia: Human Kinetics
57A Price Avenue
Lower Mitcham, South Australia 5062
08 8372 0999
e-mail: info@hkaustralia.com

New Zealand: Human Kinetics
P.O. Box 80
Torrens Park, South Australia 5062
0800 222 062
e-mail: info@hknewzealand.com

E5093

CONTENTS

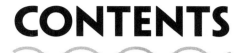

PART II   **DEEP-WATER EXERCISE**   **99**

PREFACE

In 2003, 1.9 million people were participating in water fitness, and that number keeps growing. People have been exercising in the water at least since the 1930s (United States Water Fitness Association [USWFA], 2007). Early participants were mainly older adults and special populations. Water fitness continues to appeal to baby boomers, but the market has grown to include recreational athletes, professional and elite athletes, younger adults, mind–body enthusiasts, and "prehab" clients, who are undertaking physical conditioning to prepare for surgery. Although women have been the predominant demographic for water fitness classes, that is changing as more men become involved, especially in personal training sessions. Facilities are trying to boost revenue by increasing their aquatic fitness programming to include additional formats. There is a high demand for instructors to teach these classes, but facilities report that good instructors are hard to find.

Aquatic certifications have been offered since the 1980s (USWFA, 2007; Young Men's Christian Association [YMCA], 2000). These certifications give new instructors important basic information, but instructors still have to come up with their own ideas for how to organize their classes. Often they teach their favorite exercises in whatever order occurs to them at the time, until they settle on something that seems to work well. They then repeat that routine for all of their classes. Even experienced instructors sometimes find themselves in a rut, teaching the same routines over and over again. Continuing education training, which can provide fresh ideas, is available in some large markets, but it is not available everywhere. The purpose of *Water Fitness Lesson Plans and Choreography* is to bridge that gap.

This book provides all the information about lesson plans that I wish I had when I was starting out as a new instructor. It explains class objectives, the warm-up, the conditioning phase, and the cool-down as well as the purpose of each. It describes two strategies for organizing the conditioning phase if your class objective is cardiorespiratory fitness, and how to teach a circuit class if your objective is muscular strength and endurance. It takes the mystery out of choreography by describing four choreography styles that are easy to use and easy to remember. The troubleshooting tips were gleaned from years of teaching experience. This book clarifies the differences between shallow-water exercise and deep-water exercise. The exercise lists include both common names for the exercises and their anatomical movement terms as well as which muscles are most involved. Mastering anatomical movement terms such as *abduction* and *adduction* can be challenging for new instructors, and putting the terms together with exercise names simplifies the process. Understanding which muscles you are working is important for developing balanced workouts.

Water Fitness Lesson Plans and Choreography gives you practical information for translating your technical training into usable lesson plans. This book includes 36 shallow-water lesson plans and 36 corresponding deep-water lesson plans so you can avoid getting stuck in a tired routine. It is divided into two parts, the first part dealing with shallow-water exercise and the second dealing with deep-water exercise.

The first part will help you determine what your class objective is and explain the purpose of each of the three parts of every water fitness class. It has suggestions for classes that focus on cardiorespiratory fitness and for those that focus on muscular strength and endurance so that you can help your participants meet the recommendations of the American College of Sports Medicine in a variety of ways. Using the various choreography styles will keep your classes interesting. I include information about modifying your class for various populations, choosing music, and making pre-class preparations, as well as for dealing with some of the problems and surprises that might crop up while you are teaching. Descriptions and photos of the exercises used in shallow water and which muscles are used are followed by 36 lesson plans.

The second part deals with deep-water exercise. It includes a chapter containing information specific to deep water to help you meet the challenges of teaching deep-water classes. Descriptions and photos of the exercises and which muscles are used are followed by 36 lesson plans. Because deep-water exercise is very different from shallow-water exercise, not all of the exercises are the same, but the lesson plans are similar to the shallow-water lesson plans. That way, if you have to teach a shallow-water class followed by a deep-water class, you can use, for example, Shallow-Water Lesson Plan 5: Circuit Workout 1 for the first class, and Deep-Water Lesson Plan 5: Circuit Workout 1 for the second class. All you have to remember are the specific modifications for your deep-water class.

The tools provided in this book will help you understand the purpose behind everything you teach in your classes. This will make you just the kind of good instructor aquatic facilities are looking for!

REFERENCES

USWFA. (2007). *National Water Fitness Instructors Manual*. Boynton Beach, FL: United States Water Fitness Association.

YMCA. (2000). *YMCA Water Fitness for Health*. Champaign, IL: Human Kinetics.

ACKNOWLEDGMENTS

I would like to give special thanks to the following people:
My husband, Jim, whose love and moral support were constant and whose computer knowledge kept this project from derailing on numerous occasions.

My son Adam, whose expertise as a personal trainer was invaluable in helping me understand and describe the biomechanics of the exercises.

Rotha Crump, a gracious mentor during my early experiences as a water fitness instructor, who always takes the time to answer my questions.

Anne Hensarling, the coordinator at Oak Point Recreation Center where I teach water fitness classes, who not only is a pleasure to work for but also made it possible for us to have the photo shoot at the pool.

Natasha Robalik, who challenges me to step outside my comfort zone and take on projects that have expanded my knowledge and experience in the field of water fitness.

My models, Johnnene Addison-Gay, Adam Alexander, Kathy Bolla, Rita Bryant, Anne Hensarling, and Amos Maxie, who did a professional job of performing the exercises for the photographs.

James Wiseman, the photographer who did a wonderful job, both on the deck and underwater.

The staff of Oak Point Recreation Center in Plano, Texas, who cheerfully made numerous adjustments in their routines and the pool schedule so that we could conduct the photo shoot there.

The participants in my classes who let me try out all of my lesson plans and choreography and who offer me lots of feedback.

Gayle Kassing and Amy Stahl, my editors, and the staff at Human Kinetics, whose experience and encouragement in making this book a reality are very much appreciated.

PART I

SHALLOW-WATER EXERCISE

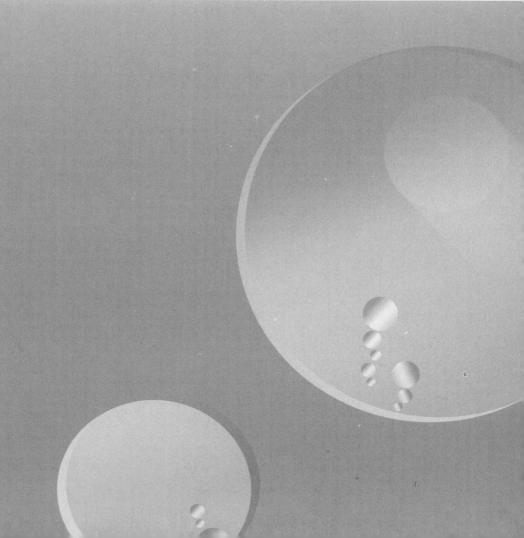

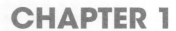

Introduction to Shallow-Water Exercise

It's show time! Your first water fitness class is an exciting event. You may have taken a water fitness instructor course or gotten a national certification. You know where your trapezius is, you have figured out the difference between abduction and adduction, and you remember that the target heart rate for cardiorespiratory training is between 60 and 80 percent of the maximum heart rate. Now you have a class to teach! You want to make a good impression. You want to lead your participants in an effective workout, and you want them to come back for the next class. How do you use what you have learned in your certification course to organize your class?

PREPARING YOUR CLASS

Your class will be most successful if you plan ahead. Begin by thinking about what you are trying to accomplish in your class time. This is your class objective, your goal for your participants. You will build your plan for the class around this objective. Your class plan will include a warm-up phase, a conditioning phase, and a cool-down phase.

DETERMINING YOUR CLASS OBJECTIVE

The first step in planning for any water fitness class is to decide what your objective is. The class description in your facility brochure may state your objective. If the name of your class is Hydro Cardio Fit or Power Splash Dance (USWFA, 2007), then you know the participants coming to your class will be expecting cardiorespiratory fitness training. Often the objective is left up to the instructor. The two most common objectives are cardiorespiratory fitness and muscular strength and endurance. It is also possible to do both in the same class.

The second step in planning your class is to write a lesson plan that meets your class objective. A lesson plan is a list of the exercises you plan to use in your class. When choosing your exercises, keep in mind the three parts of every class—the warm-up, the conditioning phase, and the cool-down (Aquatic Exercise Association [AEA], 2006).

WARM-UP PHASE

The average temperature of the water in an indoor multipurpose pool is 84 to 86 degrees Fahrenheit (29 to 30 °C) (USWFA, 2007). Your average body temperature is 98.6 degrees Fahrenheit (37 °C). This means that the pool temperature will be 12 to 14 degrees (around 7 °C) cooler than your body, and it always feels cold when you first get in the water. The purpose of the first part of your warm-up is to adjust participants' body temperatures to the water temperature. A vigorous, short-lever move, such as a knee-high jog, works well to start out the warm-up. Don't forget to cue good posture! As the water begins to feel more comfortable to participants, you can start to have them warm up their muscles and increase their heart rates in preparation for the workout. Use moves to the front, the sides, and the back of the body to make sure all the muscles warm up. Progress from short-lever moves to longer-lever moves. The entire warm-up should take between 5 and 10 minutes.

One way to have participants warm up is to have them jog in place for two to three minutes; then water walk the length of the pool and back. They should walk forward, backward, and sideways. Another idea is to have them do some light jogging with various arm moves. Have them use a knee-high jog, a straddle jog, and a heel jog to use different leg muscles as they warm up the upper body. You can also use the warm-up to introduce moves you are going to use in the conditioning phase that may be new to your participants. Have them begin with a knee-high jog; then introduce the new moves at half speed, increasing to regular water tempo as they catch on. The following two sample warm-ups will get you started.

FIVE-MINUTE WARM-UP

Kick forward with shoulder blade squeeze (1 min.)

Knee-high jog, palms touch in back (30 secs.)

Run tires, reach to the sides (30 secs.)

Rocking horse to the right side (30 secs.)

Kick side to side (30 secs.)

Rocking horse to the left side (30 secs.)

Jumping jacks (30 secs.)

In-line skate (30 secs.)

Skate kick (30 secs.)

TEN-MINUTE WARM-UP

Knee-high jog with jog press (1 min.)

Knee-high jog with shoulder blade squeeze (1 min.)

Straddle jog, palms touch in front (1 min.)

Straddle jog, palms touch in back (1 min.)

Kick side to side (30 secs.)

Ankle touch (30 secs.)

Hopscotch (30 secs.)

Jumping jacks (30 secs.)

Jacks tuck (30 secs.)

Tuck ski (30 secs.)

Cross-country ski (30 secs.)

Rocking horse right, travel backward (45 secs.)

Rocking horse left, travel forward (45 secs.)

Rocking horse right, travel sideways (30 secs.)

Rocking horse left, travel sideways (30 secs.)

By the end of the warm-up, the water will feel comfortable or even slightly warm to your participants, they will be breathing a bit harder, and their muscles will be ready for the increased intensity of the conditioning phase.

CONDITIONING PHASE

The conditioning phase is the main section of your class, and it takes up the major portion of your class time. Your participants are there for a workout to maintain or improve their current level of physical fitness. Two of the components of physical fitness are cardiorespiratory endurance, and muscular strength and endurance (USWFA, 2007). The conditioning phase focuses on one or both of these components. Improving cardiorespiratory endurance means improving the ability of the heart and lungs to deliver oxygen to the working muscles (USWFA, 2007). The American College of Sports Medicine recommends moderately intense cardio work for 30 minutes a day, five days a week, or vigorously intense cardio work for 20 minutes a day, three days a week to accomplish this goal (American College of Sports Medicine [ACSM], 2007). To improve muscular strength and endurance, you must overload the muscles to the point that you achieve gains in the amount of force you can exert and improve your ability to exert force repeatedly (USWFA, 2007). The American College of Sports Medicine recommends 8 to 10 strength training exercises, with 8 to 12 repetitions of each exercise, twice a week to accomplish this goal (ACSM, 2007). Keep the recommendations of the American College of Sports Medicine in mind when you design the conditioning phase of your lesson plans.

Conditioning Phase: Cardiorespiratory Fitness

Maximum heart rate is determined by using the formula 220 minus age (USWFA, 2007). For cardiorespiratory fitness, a heart rate of between 60 and 80 percent of maximum heart rate is considered appropriate (AEA, 2006). This range is referred to as the target heart rate (USWFA, 2007). Participants who want to do moderately intense cardio work, work out in the lower level of the target heart rate, and those who want to do vigorously intense cardio work, work out in the upper level of the target heart rate. New instructors are taught how to use the talk test and Borg's rating of perceived exertion scale to judge whether their participants are working at their target heart rates. Both of these methods are subjective but fairly accurate (AEA, 2006). If your participants want to know their exact heart rates, they need to use a heart rate monitor. A heart rate chart such as the one in table 1.1 can give them an idea of what their target heart rates should be.

The heart rate chart in table 1.1 takes into account the fact that the human heart has an estimate of seven beats per minute fewer in shallow water than on land. Heart rates are lower in water than on land, although the exercise intensity is the same. Various theories have been postulated to explain this. Certain medications and the fitness level of the participant also affect heart rate. Therefore, heart rate

TABLE 1.1

Target Heart Rates in Shallow Water

Formula: [(220 − age) × % intensity] − 7

Age	% INTENSITY						
	55%	60%	65%	70%	75%	80%	85%
25	100	110	120	130	139	149	159
30	98	107	117	126	136	145	155
35	95	104	113	123	132	141	150
40	92	101	110	119	128	137	146
45	89	98	107	116	124	133	142
50	87	95	104	112	121	129	138
55	84	92	100	109	117	125	133
60	81	89	97	105	113	121	129
65	78	86	94	102	109	117	125
70	76	83	91	98	106	113	121
75	73	80	87	95	102	109	116
80	70	77	84	91	98	105	112

charts are not accurate for everyone and should be used only to establish general guidelines.

Target heart rates are achieved by working large-muscle groups continuously and rhythmically. The two options for meeting the objective of training for cardiorespiratory fitness are a continuous training format and an interval training format.

Continuous Training Format.   In continuous training, you bring your participants up to their target heart rates and have them remain there for the duration of the conditioning phase. The conditioning phase should last at least 30 minutes to meet the American College of Sports Medicine's recommendations for moderate physical activity (ACSM, 2007). Your class should include exercises that use large-muscle groups continuously and rhythmically. Save exercises such as upper-body moves in a lunge position, lower-body moves seated on a noodle, and balance exercises for the cool-down portion of your class because they bring the heart rate down. The best way to see if your exercise selection is appropriate is to practice the moves yourself ahead of time wearing a heart rate monitor.

Interval Training Format.   In interval training, you bring your participants up to the lower or midlevel of their target heart rates. Then you periodically increase the intensity so that their heart rates climb into the upper level of their target heart rates for a short time before decreasing the intensity to let the heart rates go back into the mid- or lower level. Interval training is great for improving cardiorespiratory fitness. The two things you need to know to lead an interval class are how to increase and decrease intensity, and how long to have participants work in the upper level of the target heart rate.

Following are six factors you can address to increase intensity in shallow water:

1. Speed
2. Range of motion
3. Suspended moves
4. Power
5. Travel
6. Rebound

Increasing speed effectively results in performing the move faster without compromising range of motion. Often participants go faster but make the move smaller. Encourage them not to go so fast that they find themselves doing tiny moves at top speed because this is not an effective way to increase intensity. Increasing range of motion involves performing exercises with long levers (arms and legs slightly flexed) through their full range of motion. In suspended moves, participants pick up their feet and perform the moves without touching the bottom of the pool. Increasing power is about pushing harder against the resistance of the water. Travel involves moving through the water from one part of the pool to another. Participants can achieve some of their highest intensity levels by traveling through the water at maximum speed. They can travel forward, backward, or sideways. Rebounding means jumping. Some younger participants love to jump, but older adults, obese participants, and people with hip, knee, or feet issues should not rebound. If you choose to increase intensity by using rebounding, offer options for those who should avoid jumping, such as performing the same move in a neutral position with the hips and knees flexed and the shoulders at the surface of the water (AEA, 2006). In the lesson plans in this book, the exercises used to bring the heart rate up during interval sessions are labeled *interval high-intensity phase*.

To decrease intensity, participants can slow down, decrease their range of motion, allow their feet to touch the floor following a suspended move, ease back from the power moves, perform the exercise in place, or drop back from rebounding to a move that keeps one foot on the floor. In the lesson plans with intervals in this book, the exercises used to decrease heart rate following the high-intensity phase are labeled *interval active recovery phase*.

Timing the Intervals. How long you work your class in the upper level of the target heart rate depends on the fitness levels of your participants. A simple plan is to have them work in the lower to midlevel of their target heart rates for eight or nine minutes; then work really hard for one or two minutes. The cycle is then repeated three times in a 30-minute conditioning set or four times in a 40-minute conditioning set. You can shorten the cycle all the way down to four minutes in the lower to midlevel of the target heart rate with one minute of high-intensity work so that participants complete six cycles in a 30-minute conditioning set or eight cycles in a 40-minute conditioning set.

Some participants have difficulty working at a high intensity for one continuous minute. These participants can work in the lower to midlevel of their target heart rate for five to nine minutes, and then work really hard for 20 seconds, take a 10-second break during which they back off the intensity a little, and repeat.

They can repeat the cycle of 20 seconds of work followed by 10 seconds of active recovery two to four times. You can also play with the length of the work-and-active-recovery cycle depending on the abilities of your participants, or just to add variety. Try 30 seconds of work to 15 seconds of active recovery, or 45 seconds of work to 30 seconds of active recovery. The active recovery stage can also be longer than the work stage; for example, 45 seconds of work and 60 seconds of active recovery, or 30 seconds of work and 45 to 60 seconds of active recovery. The form and the duration of interval training have been left up to you in the lesson plans using intervals in this book.

Conditioning Phase: Muscular Strength and Endurance

If your objective is muscular strength and endurance training, keep in mind that participants will tend to get chilled while remaining stationary and focusing on working with resistance unless they are in a warm-water pool. Because most recreational pools are not warm-water pools, you will want to intersperse strength training exercises with periods of moving around to keep the muscles warm. Participants need to overload their muscles with some kind of resistance for the exercise to be effective. They can do this without equipment by pushing hard against the resistance of the water. The more force they use, the greater the resistance (YMCA, 2000). They can also use arm moves or leg moves that pull the body either forward or backward while traveling in the opposite direction. For example, they can do a breaststroke, which pulls the body forward, while traveling backward.

Another option is to add equipment. Many facilities have noodles or foam dumbbells, and some participants like to bring their own webbed gloves. Avoid doing an entire class with foam dumbbells, though, because that puts too much strain on the shoulder joint. Alternate upper-body strength training using noodles for resistance with lower-body strength training using noodles for flotation. Participants can keep warm by traveling while doing the upper-body strength training.

Circuit Format.　The circuit format is one of the most popular ways to do muscular strength and endurance training in the water. A typical circuit class has stations set up around the edge of the pool. Place a sign with the name of a strength training exercise at each station; then lead your class in a few rhythmic exercises to keep their muscles warm. Next, have participants go to a station and do the exercise described on the sign. They can divide up among the stations, or they can all go from station to station as a group. If they are going from station to station as a group, the signs are not essential.

You may have different types of equipment at each station, but this is not required. A circuit class that alternates rhythmic exercise sets to keep warm and strength training sets without equipment is sometimes called a modified circuit class. Because facilities vary widely in the type of equipment they have on hand, this book includes only one circuit lesson plan that uses dumbbells, but they are optional. Feel free to use whatever equipment you have available, but make sure you know how to use the equipment before you try it out on your class.

Core Strength Training.　You may want to teach a class that focuses on core strength. See Shallow-Water Lesson Plan 9: Core Challenge. Working out in the water is great for improving core strength because the properties of water are constantly challenging balance. You can increase the challenge for the core muscles by having participants balance on one foot and work the other leg, perform suspended moves and log jumps, work only one arm, or travel without using their arms to assist balance.

Combining Cardiorespiratory Fitness and Strength Training. You can get the best of both worlds by incorporating strength training into an interval class, creating a workout that has both cardiorespiratory fitness and muscular strength and endurance as its objective. Combine upper-body moves with aerobic exercises to bring your participants up to the lower or midlevel of their target heart rates. In this case, the overload for strength training comes from pushing hard against the water or from using webbed gloves.

Every 5 to 10 minutes during the conditioning phase, increase the intensity using speed, range of motion, suspended moves, power, travel, or rebounding as described earlier so that the heart rate climbs into the upper level of the target heart rate for a short time before decreasing the intensity to let the heart rate go back into the mid- or lower level. It is a good idea to include exercises for the upper body in your cardio classes even when muscular strength and endurance is not your class objective. You can have participants do arm exercises while performing leg moves or add an arm medley with a knee-high jog.

Conditioning Phase: Choreography Options

Your lesson plan is a list of the exercises you plan to use in your class. Choreography is the way you organize those exercises to give them logic and flow and make them easy to remember. Choreography can be as simple as a list of exercises with no repetitions, or as complicated as planning specific moves to go with the lyrics of a song or a piece of music. The choreography in this book is designed to be easy for you to teach and your participants to follow. As you gain experience, you may wish to write your own choreography and experiment with more complex patterns. The four strategies for developing choreography are linear choreography, variations on a theme, add-on choreography, and block choreography. Variations on a theme is a form of linear choreography.

Linear Choreography. In linear choreography, the exercises are written in a list from beginning to end, with no (or very little) repetition. The order of the linear choreography exercises in this book has a logical flow to help you remember what comes next. For example, in Shallow-Water Lesson Plan 1: Basic Moves, the flow is in the way the legs work from front to side to back. Cycles of four minutes of traveling are followed by one minute of strength training in Shallow-Water Lesson Plan 7: Circuit Workout 3. Similar types of exercises are grouped into sets in Shallow-Water Lesson Plan 8: Singles and Doubles.

The choreography called variations on a theme is a type of linear choreography that involves multiple variations of two or three exercises. Examples include adding different arm moves; increasing speed; taking the exercise down to a neutral position, then suspending it, and then taking it back up to rebounding; moving the legs across the body or out to the side; combining the move with another move; or traveling forward, backward, and sideways. By the end of the class you have increased and decreased intensity many times.

Add-On Choreography. Add-on choreography is a favorite of many instructors and easy to write for yourself. You put together five to seven sets with four to six exercises in each set. You teach your class the first and second sets, and then you repeat them and add the third set. You then have them repeat the first three sets and add the fourth set, and so on until they have completed all of your sets. The number of sets you need depends partly on whether you include traveling, which may take longer than stationary exercises.

Block Choreography. In block choreography, you set up a pattern in your first set that you repeat with variations in each succeeding set. For example, Shallow-Water Lesson Plan 26: Intervals With Knee-High Jog begins the first set with a stationary upper-body move followed by a traveling upper-body move. Travel continues with cross-country ski and jumping jacks. In three exercises the legs move to the sides. Finally, there are intervals with a knee-high jog that increase intensity using speed. The pattern repeats using different upper-body moves, each set focusing on a different muscle group. In sets 1 and 3 participants travel backward and forward with cross-country ski and jumping jacks, and in sets 2 and 4 they travel sideways. The sets always end with intervals with a knee-high jog, but the intensity variable changes each time.

The possible combinations and variations are endless. You may want some moves to stay the same in each set while you vary other moves. Block choreography works especially well with intervals because each set has the same number of exercises so your periods of higher intensity are spaced evenly throughout your conditioning set.

The conditioning phase is the most important part of your class, and you have many options! You can choose between the two class objectives of cardiorespiratory fitness and muscular strength and endurance, or you can combine both into one class. If you choose to focus on cardiorespiratory fitness, you can use a continuous training format or an interval format. If you choose to focus on muscular strength and endurance, you can have participants overload the muscles without equipment by pushing hard against the resistance of the water, or you can have them use equipment. You can try a circuit format, or you can combine the objectives of cardiorespiratory fitness and muscular strength and endurance in an interval class. You can also organize your lesson plans into four different choreography styles. With all these ideas, it is easy to keep your participants—and yourself—interested and challenged. Once your participants have completed the conditioning phase, it is time to begin the cool-down.

COOL-DOWN PHASE

The cool-down allows participants to slowly recover from the work they have done in the conditioning phase. If your last set ended with an interval, you will want to continue the active recovery exercise for a few minutes. Then you can have participants begin to go into slower, lower-intensity movements. One way to do this is to repeat the warm-up, perhaps in reverse order. Another option is to include a set of toning exercises. These can be exercises for muscular strength, or they can be abdominal and core strength exercises.

Because flexibility is also important, finish the cool-down with at least five minutes of stretching. Participants can do static stretches for the major muscles they worked during the class, holding each stretch for 10 to 30 seconds. If participants get chilled standing motionless holding a stretch, have them do dynamic stretching instead, moving their muscles slowly through their full range of motion. You can also include yoga poses and Ai Chi, if you are familiar with those forms of exercise and how to adapt them to the water. Tai Chi that is adapted for water fitness is called Ai Chi.

MODIFYING YOUR LESSON PLAN FOR DIFFERENT POPULATIONS

You should not assume that everyone in your class has the same fitness level that you have. Neither should you assume that just because your participants are older, they need a gentle workout. Observe your participants to see what they are capable of, and teach to those capabilities. Offer options for those who want a higher intensity level as well as options for those who need a lower intensity level from the rest of the class. For example, you could teach a frog jump in the neutral position and then give your participants the option to take it up to a rebound. Offer a straddle jog to participants who need to work at a lower intensity.

In general, older adults need a longer warm-up to allow time for their joints to warm up. Avoid jumping and instead offer low-impact options. Include movements that change direction to improve balance and coordination. Also include muscular strengthening and stretching exercises (AEA, 2006).

If your class includes men, avoid cute dance moves. Instead, use callisthenic-type moves such as jumping jacks and cross-country ski. Keep your choreography simple, and have participants stay with a move for at least eight repetitions or longer before changing to another move. Men are often unwilling to participate in partner moves. Circuit classes and classes with muscular strength and endurance as their objective work well.

You may have participants in your class who have arthritis. Many people with mild to moderate arthritis do well in regular fitness classes. Participants with moderate to severe arthritis may be better served in an arthritis class. Contact the Arthritis Foundation (www.arthritis.org) to take their certification class if you wish to be involved in these types of classes.

Cardiac patients, disabled people, and rehab patients need guidance from a doctor or a physical therapist. Working with athletes requires special training. Be sure you are qualified before taking on special populations that require skills beyond those taught in a typical certification class.

MUSIC

Your next step in preparing to teach your class is to decide whether to use music. Sometimes there is so much activity going on in the pool during your class that you may choose not to add another layer to the noise level. Sometimes participants will be able to hear your voice better if you are not competing with music. On the other hand, many instructors and their participants enjoy the motivation that comes from music. Before choosing your music, remember that U.S. copyright laws state that copyright owners have the right to charge a fee for the use of their music in public performances. Water fitness classes are considered public performances (AEA, 2006). Therefore, use music that is produced by businesses that pay the copyright fees and not music that you have recorded yourself. Music that is 130 to 145 beats per minute works well for shallow-water exercise and with all of the shallow-water choreography in this book.

TEACHING YOUR CLASS

Always arrive early to check out the pool before your class. What area of the pool will your participants be using? If you are using equipment, where is it located? If you are using music, where is the music player kept? Where are the locker rooms? Are there any tripping hazards between the locker room and the pool that you need to clear out of the way? Is the pool deck wet or slippery? Where will you stand when you teach your class? Whether to teach on the deck or in the water is a subject of great debate among water fitness instructors. Whichever you choose to do, make sure your participants will be able to see and hear you and understand your cues. Often the deck surface is concrete. Wear good, supportive water fitness shoes. If you choose to teach from the deck, or to teach part of the time from the deck and part of the time in the pool, ask the facility to provide a mat, and use it. You want to protect yourself from developing feet, knee, or hip injuries. With your lesson plan ready and your pool space as safe as you can make it, you are ready to greet your participants.

TROUBLESHOOTING

- **What should you do if you get to the end of your lesson plan and there are still 10 minutes of class left?** It takes practice to get your timing down. Fill up those 10 minutes by repeating the warm-up or the first set or by adding extra strength training or abdominal exercises at the end of class.

- **What should you do if some of your participants don't seem to be able to follow your cues?** Allow your participants to perform each exercise at least eight times before moving on to the next exercise, at least the first time around. Some people will not be able to keep up if you pace the exercises too quickly. If that doesn't solve the problem, try using a variety of cueing techniques. Cues can be visual or audible. Visual cues include physical demonstrations and hand signals. Audible cues include spoken instruction, hand claps, and whistles (AEA, 2006). Consider using a deck microphone if possible. Cues can also be physical, such as pointing to the muscle you want your participant to focus on, but never touch anyone without permission.

- **What should you do if a participant is performing an exercise incorrectly?** Make sure you are demonstrating the exercise with good form. You may want to stand closer to your participant so she can have a better view of how you are doing the exercise, but don't single out an individual for correction in front of the class. Instead, cue a reminder of proper form to the entire class.

- **What should you do if a participant is not following your directions?** It is not uncommon to have a participant who does not put much effort into the workout, or who always seems to be doing an exercise different from the one you are cueing. He may have some kind of physical issue that he has not told you about, such as arthritis or an injury. Give him the benefit of the doubt and assume that he is doing the best he can.

- **What should you do if one of your participants asks you a medical question?** Always know your limitations. Don't give medical advice. Refer your participant back to her own doctor.

- **What should you do if some of your participants are spending more time talking with each other than exercising?** This might be a good time to teach in the pool. Circulate among your participants and give them some individual encouragement, especially the talkers. Often this is all that is needed to get them more involved in the class. Sometimes, however, participants come to a class for the social aspects. If this is their objective, then you just need to have patience with them.

- **What should you do if one of your participants is afraid of water?** Suggest that he work close to the wall in the shallowest part of the pool. You can give him a noodle to hold on to for added stability. Tell him that he does not have to travel until he feels comfortable doing so. Do not allow him to hang from the wall with his back to the wall and his elbows on the deck because this has the potential of injuring the shoulder joints (AEA, 2006). Often, after a few classes, such participants begin to overcome their fear of water.

- **What should you do if some of your participants are afraid to pick their feet up off the floor for suspended moves?** Offer them options in the neutral position, such as performing the move faster, increasing the range of motion, or adding power. You may also need to be prepared to offer abdominal exercises that can be done in a standing position such as pelvic tilts, standing crunches, and balance moves. Participants who are afraid to pick their feet up off the floor are often uncomfortable floating on a noodle as well.

- **What should you do if some of your participants don't seem to be working very hard during suspended moves?** Some participants work very hard to stay suspended. But others float easily and for them suspended moves do not increase their heart rates. In that case, offer them options that will make the move harder, such as working suspended at a faster speed, using longer levers, adding power, and traveling while suspended.

- **What should you do if your participants fill up the space in the pool and there is not enough room for traveling?** This problem has more solutions than you might imagine. Consider the following:

    1. Have participants perform an exercise four times and then turn to the left side of the pool; perform the exercise four times and then face the back of the pool; perform the exercise four times and turn to the right side of the pool; and perform the exercise four times and turn to face you. This is called a quarter turn.

    2. Have participants perform an exercise four times traveling backward and four times traveling forward, continuing to travel back and forth. The quick change of direction challenges balance and core muscles.

    3. Divide the participants into two groups facing each other on opposite sides of the pool. Have them travel forward to the opposite side of the pool to change places.

    4. Gather participants in a big circle and have them travel a few steps toward the center of the circle and a few steps back, or clockwise and counterclockwise. Do not have them travel any great distance clockwise or counterclockwise, though, because a current quickly forms that can sweep some participants off their feet.

5. To avoid creating a current, divide your participants into two concentric circles. The inner circle might travel clockwise, and the outer circle, counterclockwise. The turbulence created by this pattern also challenges core muscles.

6. If you have something similar to four lap lanes, divide the class into two groups. One group travels down the first lap lane and up the second lap lane, and the other group travels down the third lap lane and up the fourth lap lane. The effect will be travel in two oval patterns side by side.

7. Have participants travel in a scatter pattern, over all parts of the pool area.

PUTTING IT ALL TOGETHER

You now have some tools for beginning your career as a water fitness instructor. You understand that every class has an objective and that the two most common objectives are cardiorespiratory fitness and muscular strength and endurance. You know about the three parts of every class—the warm-up, the conditioning phase, and the cool-down. You have some ideas for designing the warm-up. You know how to use a continuous training format and an interval format when your class objective is cardiorespiratory fitness. You have some ideas for how to increase and decrease intensity to help your participants work in their target heart rates. You have information on how to overload the muscles when your objective is muscular strength and endurance, and how to use a circuit format. You also have learned how to combine both objectives in one class. You have options for organizing the exercises into logical patterns using linear choreography, variations on a theme, add-on choreography, and block choreography. You understand how to use the cool-down to allow your participants to slowly recover from the conditioning phase and then stretch. You have some suggestions for modifying your lesson plan for various populations and suggestions for using music. You have some tips for your pre-class preparations and for troubleshooting when the unexpected happens. Now you are ready for a look at the exercises and cueing tips in chapter 2.

REFERENCES

ACSM. (2007). *Physical Activity and Public Health Guidelines*. Retrieved August 20, 2009, from American College of Sports Medicine: www.acsm.org//AM/Template.cfm?Section=Home_Page.

AEA. (2006). *Aquatic Fitness Professional Manual*. Champaign, IL: Human Kinetics.

USWFA. (2007). *National Water Fitness Instructors Manual*. Boynton Beach, FL: United States Water Fitness Association.

YMCA. (2000). *YMCA Water Fitness for Health*. Champaign, IL: Human Kinetics.

Shallow-Water Exercises and Cueing Tips

The list of shallow-water exercises begins with exercises for cardiorespiratory fitness—walk, jog, kick, rocking horse, cross-country ski, jumping jacks, and jump, and variations of each. These are followed by strength training exercises for the upper body, abdominals, obliques, and lower body. The last group of exercises is for improving balance.

Some of these exercise groups—jog; kick; and the exercises for the upper body, abdominals, obliques, and lower body—are further divided into sub-groups, which are indicated by boldface type and italics for the title of the first exercise in each sub-group. The muscles used for each exercise and the variations are listed. At the end of each group and sub-group, the directions of travel are listed that are possible for that group of exercises. The muscles used here will be the same for the stationary exercise.

WALK

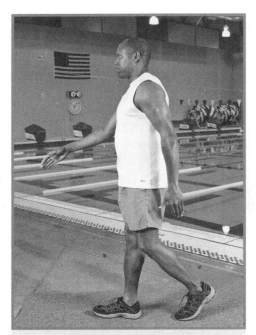

FIGURE 2.1 Walk forward: Walk with a natural arm swing.

Walk forward (hip and knee flexion and extension; see figure 2.1); *muscles used:* hip flexors, hamstrings, quadriceps

▶ **CUEING TIPS:** Walk upright with good posture. Walk forward heel-toe.

Walk backward; *muscles used:* gluteus maximus, hamstrings

▶ **CUEING TIP:** Walk backward toe-heel.

Knee lift, big step, travel forward and backward; *muscles used:* hip flexors, hamstrings, quadriceps, gluteus maximus

Walk 4×, jog 8×; *muscles used:* hip flexors, hamstrings, quadriceps

Walk on toes; *muscle used:* gastrocnemius

Walk on heels; *muscle used:* tibilias anterior

Lunge forward low in the water; *muscles used:* quadriceps, gluteus maximus

Crossover step (hip adduction; see figure 2.2); *muscles used:* hip adductors

▶ **CUEING TIP:** Step right foot over left, left foot over right.

Two steps forward, side, back, side (see figure 2.3); *muscles used:* hip flexors, hamstrings, quadriceps, gluteus medius, gluteus maximus

▶ **CUEING TIPS:** Travel in a straight line; take two steps forward, turn, take two steps sideways, turn, take two steps backward, turn, take two steps facing the other side.

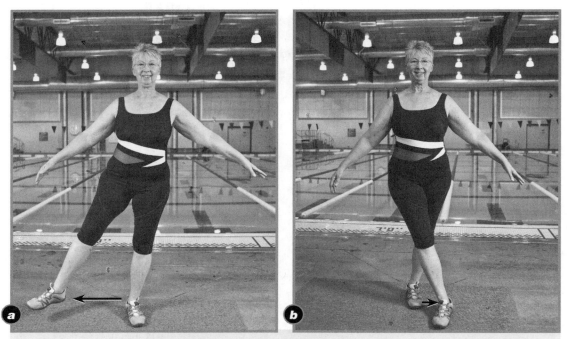

FIGURE 2.2 Crossover step: *(a)* **Abduct one leg;** *(b)* **step across the midline of the body.**

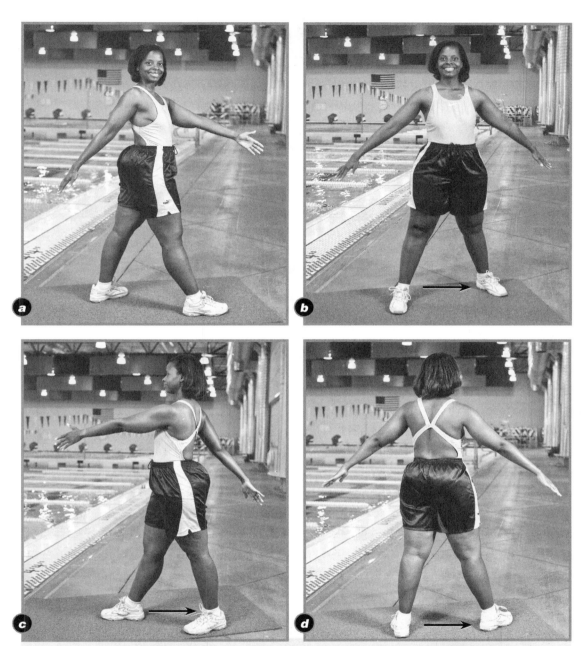

FIGURE 2.3 Two steps forward, side, back, side: *(a)* Step forward right left; *(b)* turn to the right and take two steps to the left; *(c)* turn backward and take two steps backward left right; *(d)* turn to the right and take two steps to the right.

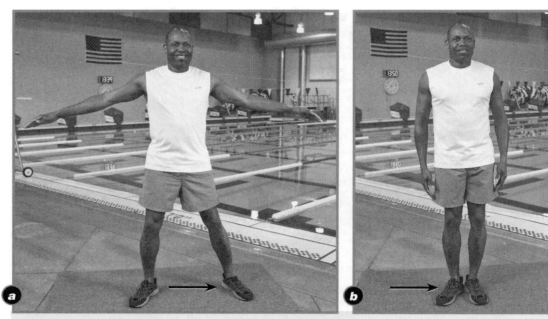

FIGURE 2.4 **Step sideways:** *(a)* **Step to the side with one leg;** *(b)* **step together with the other leg.**

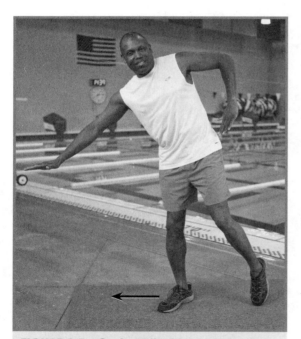

FIGURE 2.5 **Crab walk sideways: Lunge to the side; travel sideways.**

Step sideways (hip abduction; see figure 2.4); *muscles used:* gluteus medius, hip adductors

Crab walk sideways (see figure 2.5); *muscles used:* gluteus medius, obliques

▶ **CUEING TIPS:** Lunge to the side like a crab walking sideways. Lift the back elbow with each lunge step.

Knee lift, big step, travel sideways; *muscles used:* hip flexors, hamstrings, gluteus medius

Squat travel sideways; *muscles used:* gluteus maximus, hamstrings, hip flexors, quadriceps

JOG

Knee-high jog (hip and knee flexion; see figure 2.6); *muscles used:* hip flexors, hamstrings, quadriceps

▶ **CUEING TIP:** Bring the knee up to hip level; land toe-ball-heel.

Knee-high jog with or without a bounce; *muscles used:* hip flexors, hamstrings, quadriceps

Knee-high jog, neutral position; *muscles used:* hip flexors, hamstrings, quadriceps

Knee-high jog, suspended; suspended variations: bicycle or hip curl; *muscles used:* hip flexors, hamstrings, quadriceps, core stabilizers

Knee-high jog, faster; *muscles used:* hip flexors, hamstrings, quadriceps

▶ **CUEING TIP:** Don't lose your range of motion.

Sprint; *muscles used:* hip flexors, hamstrings, quadriceps

▶ **CUEING TIPS:** Use a longer stride. Pump arms from the shoulders.

Leap (see figure 2.7); *muscles used:* hip flexors, hamstrings, quadriceps, gluteus maximus

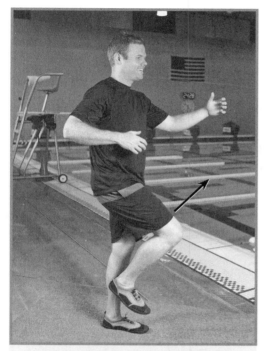

FIGURE 2.6 **Knee-high jog: Jog with the knee coming up to hip level.**

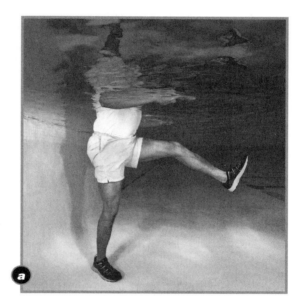

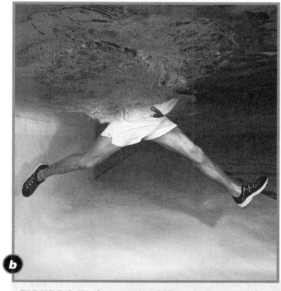

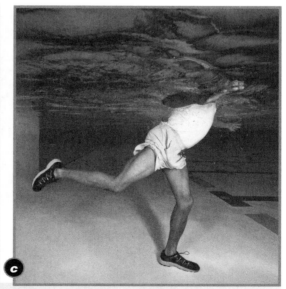

FIGURE 2.7 **Leap:** *(a)* **Lift one leg;** *(b)* **leap forward;** *(c)* **land toe-ball-heel.**

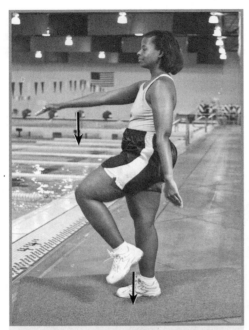

FIGURE 2.8 **Steep climb: Jog using power and power press down the arms.**

Steep climb (see figure 2.8); *muscles used:* hip flexors, hamstrings, quadriceps

▶ **CUEING TIPS:** Elbows are straight, but not locked; press down. The motion is like climbing a ladder. Use power.

Knee-high jog, one knee only; *muscles used:* hip flexors, hamstrings, quadriceps

▶ **CUEING TIP:** Hop on one foot, lift the other knee up and down.

Knee-high jog, doubles; *muscles used:* hip flexors, hamstrings, quadriceps

▶ **CUEING TIP:** Lift each knee 2×.

Skateboard (see figure 2.9); *muscles used:* hip flexors, hamstrings, quadriceps, gluteus maximus, core stabilizers

▶ **CUEING TIP:** Stand with one foot on the skateboard; pedal with the other foot.

Crossover knees (see figure 2.10); *muscles used:* hip flexors, hamstrings, quadriceps, obliques

▶ **CUEING TIP:** Hips twist, but trunk stays squared.

Knee lift and lunge (hip and knee flexion and extension); *muscles used*: hip flexors, hamstrings, quadriceps, gluteus maximus

Knee-high jog; travel forward, backward, or sideways

Sprint, travel forward

Knee-high jog with quick change of direction; *muscles used:* core stabilizers

Knee-high jog, travel in a circle

Knee-high jog, travel in a square

Knee-high jog, travel in a zigzag

Knee-high jog, travel in a scatter pattern

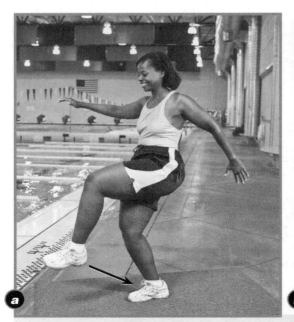
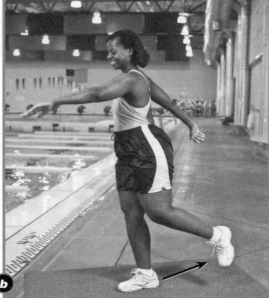

FIGURE 2.9 **Skateboard:** *(a)* **Stand on one foot;** *(b)* **pedal the other foot from front to back.**

Straddle jog (hip abduction and knee flexion; see figure 2.11); *muscles used:* gluteus medius, hip adductors, hamstrings, quadriceps

▶ **CUEING TIP:** Hips are open but feet are close together, land toe-ball-heel.

Straddle jog with or without a bounce; *muscles used:* gluteus medius, hip adductors, hamstrings, quadriceps

Straddle jog, neutral position; *muscles used:* gluteus medius, hip adductors, hamstrings, quadriceps

Straddle jog, suspended; suspended variation: diamond position, open and close knees; *muscles used:* tensor fasciae latae, hip adductors, hamstrings, quadriceps, core stabilizers

Straddle jog, faster; *muscles used:* gluteus medius, hip adductors, hamstrings, quadriceps

▶ **CUEING TIP:** Don't lose your range of motion.

Straddle jog; travel forward, backward, or sideways

Run tires (hip abduction and knee flexion; see figure 2.12); *muscles used:* gluteus medius, hip adductors, hamstrings, quadriceps

▶ **CUEING TIP:** Hips are open and feet are wide apart, land toe-ball-heel, as if running through tires at football practice.

Run tires with or without a bounce; *muscles used:* gluteus medius, hip adductors, hamstrings, quadriceps

Run tires, neutral position; *muscles used:* gluteus medius, hip adductors, hamstrings, quadriceps

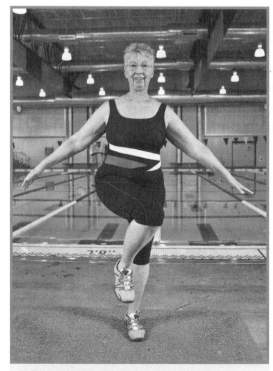

FIGURE 2.10 Crossover knees: Jog with the knee crossing the midline of the body.

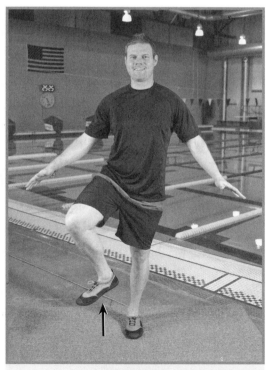

FIGURE 2.11 Straddle jog: Jog with the hips abducted and the feet under the body.

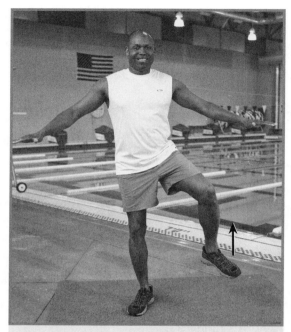

FIGURE 2.12 **Run tires: Jog with the hips abducted and the feet wide.**

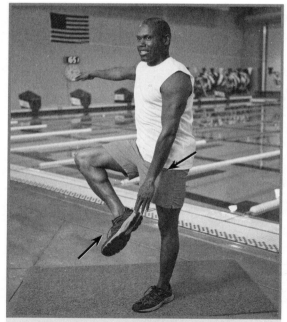

FIGURE 2.13 **Ankle touch: Touch the ankle with the opposite hand.**

Run tires, suspended; *muscles used:* tensor fasciae latae, hip adductors, hamstrings, quadriceps, core stabilizers

Run tires, faster; *muscles used:* gluteus medius, hip adductors, hamstrings, quadriceps

▶ **CUEING TIP:** Don't lose your range of motion.

Run tires, doubles; *muscles used:* gluteus medius, hip adductors, hamstrings, quadriceps

▶ **CUEING TIP:** Lift each knee 2× to the side.

In in, out out; *muscles used:* gluteus medius, hip adductors, hamstrings, quadriceps

▶ **CUEING TIP:** Jog; alternate feet in and out.

Run tires; travel forward, backward, or sideways

Ankle touch (hip flexion and lateral rotation; see figure 2.13); *muscles used:* hip flexors, tensor fasciae latae, sartorius

▶ **CUEING TIPS:** Bring the ankle up to the hand; bring the hand down to the ankle. If you can't reach the ankle, aim for the shin or knee instead.

Ankle touch with or without a bounce; *muscles used:* hip flexors, tensor fasciae latae, sartorius

Ankle touch, faster; *muscles used:* hip flexors, tensor fasciae latae, sartorius

▶ **CUEING TIP:** Don't lose your range of motion.

Ankle touch, feet close together or wide apart; *muscles used:* hip flexors, tensor fasciae latae, sartorius

Ankle touch, one ankle only; *muscles used:* hip flexors, tensor fasciae latae, sartorius

Ankle touch with double arms (see figure 2.14); *muscles used:* hip flexors, tensor fasciae latae, sartorius, core stabilizers

▶ **CUEING TIP:** Extend both arms to one side, then touch the opposite ankle with both hands.

Ankle touch, doubles

▶ **CUEING TIP:** Touch each ankle 2×.

Ankle touch, travel forward or backward

Heel jog (knee flexion; see figure 2.15); *muscles used:* hamstrings, quadriceps

▶ **CUEING TIP:** Keep knees under hips and curl the hamstrings, land toe-ball-heel.

Heel jog with or without a bounce; *muscles used:* hamstrings, quadriceps

Heel jog, faster; *muscles used:* hamstrings, quadriceps

▶ **CUEING TIP:** Don't lose your range of motion.

Heel jog, feet close together or wide apart; *muscles used:* hamstrings, quadriceps

Hitchhike (see figure 2.16); *muscles used:* hamstrings, quadriceps

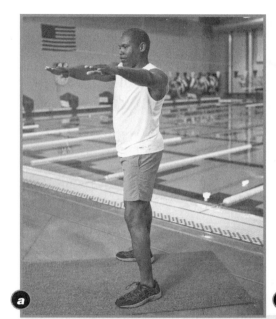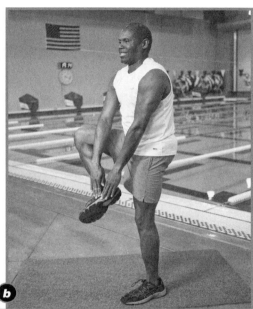

FIGURE 2.14 **Ankle touch with double arms:** *(a)* **Extend both arms to one side;** *(b)* **touch the opposite ankle with both hands.**

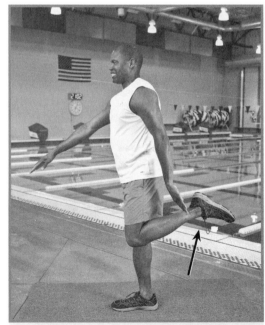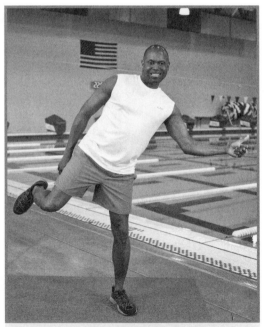

FIGURE 2.15 **Heel jog: Jog with a heel lift in back.**

FIGURE 2.16 **Hitchhike: Heel jog leaning side to side and signaling hitchhike with thumbs.**

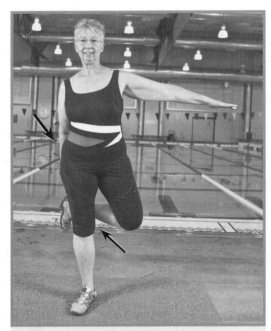

FIGURE 2.17 Hopscotch: Touch the heel in back with the opposite hand.

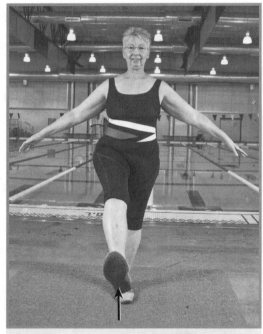

FIGURE 2.18 Kick forward: Kick forward with soft knees.

▶ **CUEING TIP:** Lean side to side lifting heels and signaling hitch-hike with thumbs.

Heel jog, one heel only; *muscles used:* hamstrings, quadriceps

▶ **CUEING TIP:** Hop on one foot and lift the other heel up and down in back.

Heel jog, doubles; *muscles used:* hamstrings, quadriceps

▶ **CUEING TIP:** Lift each heel 2×.

Heel jog; travel forward, backward, or sideways

Hopscotch (knee flexion; see figure 2.17); *muscles used:* hamstrings, quadriceps

▶ **CUEING TIPS:** Touch the heel in back with the opposite hand. If you can't touch the heel, just aim for it.

Hopscotch with or without a bounce; *muscles used:* hamstrings, quadriceps

Hopscotch, faster; *muscles used:* hamstrings, quadriceps

▶ **CUEING TIP:** Don't lose your range of motion.

Hopscotch, feet close together or wide apart; *muscles used:* hamstrings, quadriceps

Hopscotch, one heel only; *muscles used:* hamstrings, quadriceps

Hopscotch, doubles; *muscles used:* hamstrings, quadriceps

▶ **CUEING TIP:** Touch each heel 2×.

Hopscotch, travel forward or backward

KICK

Kick forward (hip flexion and knee extension; see figure 2.18); *muscles used:* hip flexors, quadriceps, hamstrings

▶ **CUEING TIP:** Keep knees soft, land toe-ball-heel.

Kick forward with or without a bounce; *muscles used:* hip flexors, quadriceps, hamstrings

Kick forward, neutral position; *muscles used:* hip flexors, quadriceps, hamstrings

Kick forward, suspended; suspended variation: seated flutter kick; *muscles used:* hip flexors, quadriceps, hamstrings, core stabilizers

Kick forward, faster; *muscles used:* hip flexors, quadriceps, hamstrings

▶ **CUEING TIP:** Don't lose your range of motion.

Small kick; *muscles used:* hip flexors, quadriceps, hamstrings

High kick; *muscles used:* hip flexors, gluteus maximus

One leg kicks forward; *muscles used:* hip flexors, gluteus maximus, core stabilizers

▶ **CUEING TIP:** Hop on one foot and lift the other leg up and down in front.

Kick forward, doubles; *muscles used:* hip flexors, quadriceps, hamstrings

▶ **CUEING TIP:** Lift each leg 2×.

Quad kick (see figure 2.19); *muscles used:* hip flexors, quadriceps, hamstrings, core stabilizers

▶ **CUEING TIP:** Hop on one foot, keep the other knee up, and kick from the knee.

Kick and lunge (knee extension, hip flexion and extension); *muscles used:* hip flexors, quadriceps, hamstrings, gluteus maximus

Chorus line kick; *muscles used:* hip flexors, quadriceps, hamstrings, core stabilizers

▶ **CUEING TIP:** Knee, down, kick, down.

Kick to the corners; *muscles used:* gluteus medius, quadriceps, hamstrings

Kick forward; travel forward, backward, or sideways

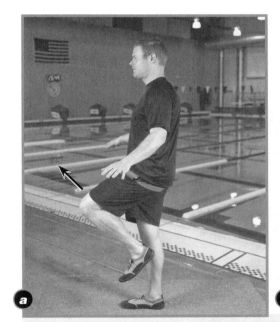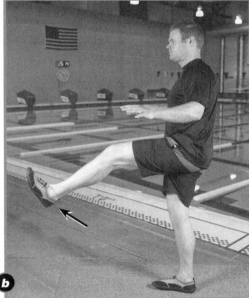

FIGURE 2.19 **Quad kick: *(a)* Lift the knee; *(b)* kick from the knee.**

Front kick (karate; see figure 2.20); *muscles used:* hip flexors, quadriceps, hamstrings

▶ **CUEING TIP:** Lift the knee and kick forward through the heel.

Skip rope (see figure 2.21); *muscles used:* hamstrings, quadriceps, hip flexors

▶ **CUEING TIP:** Heel up and kick forward.

Crossover kick (see figure 2.22); *muscles used:* hip flexors, quadriceps, hamstrings, obliques

▶ **CUEING TIP:** Kick across the body.

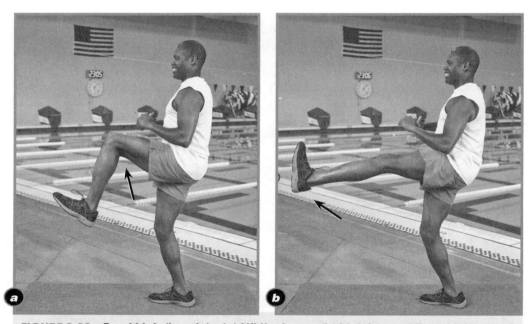

FIGURE 2.20 **Front kick (karate):** *(a)* **Lift the knee;** *(b)* **kick forward through the heel.**

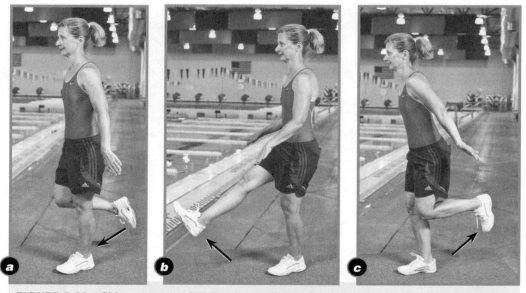

FIGURE 2.21 **Skip rope:** *(a)* **Lift the heel;** *(b)* **kick forward;** *(c)* **bring the leg down and lift the opposite heel.**

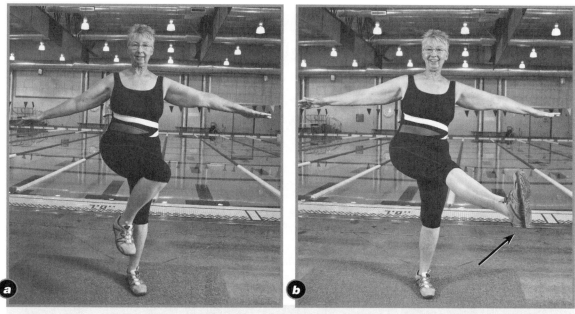

FIGURE 2.22 Crossover kick. *(a)* Lift the knee; *(b)* kick with the leg crossing the midline of the body.

Kick side to side (hip abduction; see figure 2.23); *muscles used:* gluteus medius, hip adductors

Kick side to side with or without a bounce; *muscles used:* gluteus medius, hip adductors

Kick side to side, faster; *muscles used:* gluteus medius, hip adductors

▶ **CUEING TIP:** Don't lose your range of motion.

Kick side to side, arms and legs opposite; *muscles used:* gluteus medius, hip adductors

▶ **CUEING TIP:** Use power.

One leg kicks side; *muscles used:* gluteus medius, hip adductors, core stabilizers

▶ **CUEING TIP:** Hop on one foot and lift the other leg up and down to the side.

Side quad kick (see figure 2.24); *muscles used:* gluteus medius, quadriceps, hamstrings, core stabilizers

▶ **CUEING TIP:** Hop on one foot with the other knee up to the side and kick from the knee.

Side kick (karate; see figure 2.25); *muscles used:* gluteus medius, quadriceps, hamstrings

▶ **CUEING TIP:** Lift the knee and kick to the side through the heel.

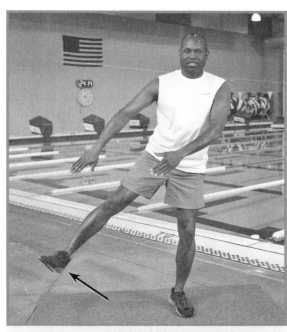

FIGURE 2.23 Kick side to side: Kick from side to side in a pendulum motion.

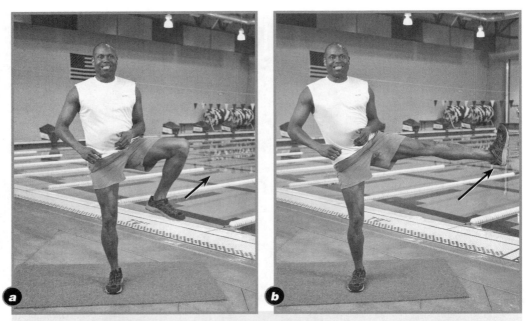

FIGURE 2.24 **Side quad kick:** *(a)* **Lift the knee to the side;** *(b)* **kick from the knee.**

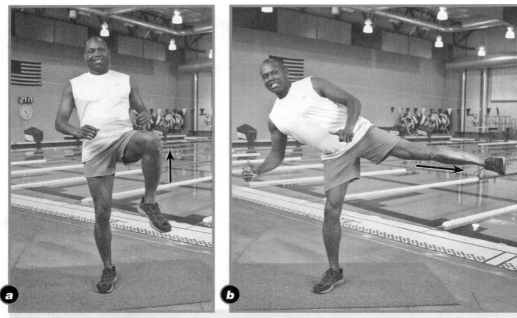

FIGURE 2.25 **Side kick (karate):** *(a)* **Lift the knee;** *(b)* **kick to the side through the heel.**

Side kick on one side, leg stays up; *muscles used:* gluteus medius, quadriceps, hamstrings, core stabilizers

Cossack kick (hip abduction and knee flexion and extension); *muscles used:* gluteus medius, quadriceps, hamstrings

▶ **CUEING TIP:** In the neutral position, feet touch the floor under the body with legs in a diamond position, and then kick to the sides.

Kick side to side; travel forward, backward, or sideways

Skate kick (hip extension; see figure 2.26); *muscle used:* gluteus maximus

▶ **CUEING TIPS:** Kick backward with the leg straight, land toe-ball-heel. Tighten the glutes.

Skate kick with or without a bounce; *muscle used:* gluteus maximus

Skate kick, faster; *muscle used:* gluteus maximus

▶ **CUEING TIP:** Don't lose your range of motion.

Skate kick, higher; *muscle used:* gluteus maximus

Skate kick with power; *muscle used:* gluteus maximus

One leg kicks back; *muscles used:* gluteus maximus, core stabilizers

▶ **CUEING TIP:** Hop on one foot and lift the other leg up and down in back.

In-line skate (see figure 2.27); *muscle used:* gluteus maximus

▶ **CUEING TIP:** Keep feet wide and step behind the opposite foot with alternating legs.

Skate kick; travel forward, backward, or sideways

Combination kicks; one leg kicks forward and back; *muscles used:* hip flexors, gluteus maximus, core stabilizers

One leg kicks forward and side; *muscles used:* hip flexors, gluteus medius, core stabilizers

One leg kicks side and back; *muscles used:* gluteus medius, gluteus maximus, core stabilizers

One leg kicks forward, side, back, side; *muscles used:* hip flexors, gluteus medius, gluteus maximus, core stabilizers

One leg—knee lift, kick forward, side knee lift, kick side, heel lift, kick back; *muscles used:* hip flexors, gluteus medius, hamstrings, gluteus maximus, core stabilizers

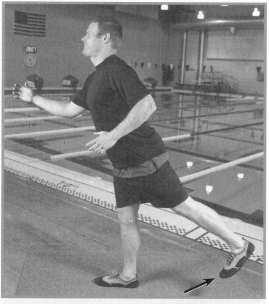

FIGURE 2.26 **Skate kick: Kick backward with the leg straight.**

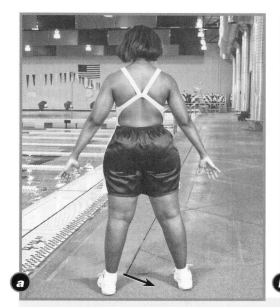 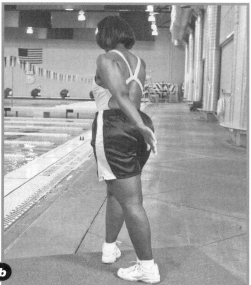

FIGURE 2.27 **In-line skate: *(a)* Begin with the feet apart; *(b)* extend the hip, stepping behind the opposite foot.**

ROCKING HORSE

Rocking horse (hip and knee flexion; see figure 2.28); *muscles used:* hip flexors, gluteus maximus, hamstrings, quadriceps

▶ **CUEING TIPS:** Rock from the front foot to the back foot. Avoid arching the back.

Rocking horse with or without a bounce; *muscles used:* hip flexors, gluteus maximus, hamstrings, quadriceps

Rocking horse, faster; *muscles used:* hip flexors, gluteus maximus, hamstrings, quadriceps

▶ **CUEING TIP:** Don't lose your range of motion.

Rocking horse to the side; *muscles used:* gluteus medius, hamstrings, quadriceps

▶ **CUEING TIP:** Hips are open, rock from side to side, knee up on one side and heel up on the other.

Rocking horse with front kick (see figure 2.29); *muscles used:* hip flexors, gluteus maximus, hamstrings, quadriceps

▶ **CUEING TIP:** Add a quad kick when you lift the knee in front.

Rocking horse; travel forward, backward, or sideways

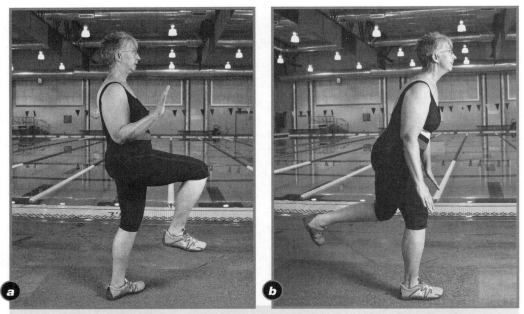

FIGURE 2.28 **Rocking horse: *(a)* Lift one knee; *(b)* bring that foot down and lift the opposite heel.**

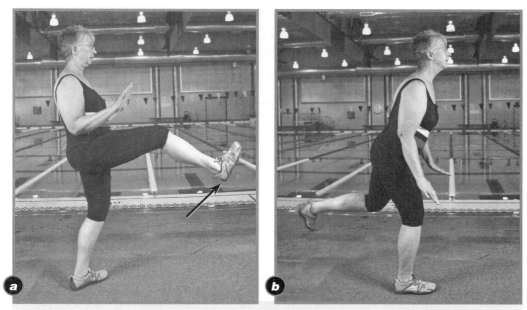

FIGURE 2.29 Rocking horse with front kick: *(a)* Lift one knee and quad kick; *(b)* bring that foot down and lift the opposite heel.

CROSS-COUNTRY SKI

Cross-country ski (hip flexion and extension; see figure 2.30); *muscles used:* gluteus maximus, hip flexors

▶ **CUEING TIP:** Start in a lunge position; then switch legs.

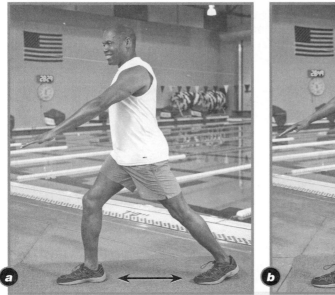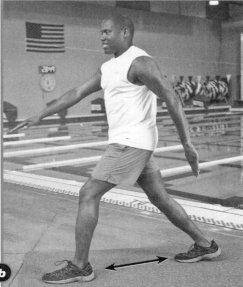

FIGURE 2.30 Cross-country ski: *(a)* Begin in a lunge position with right leg and left arm forward; *(b)* switch to the left leg and right arm forward.

Cross-country ski with or without a bounce; *muscles used:* gluteus maximus, hip flexors

Cross-country ski, neutral position; *muscles used:* gluteus maximus, hip flexors

Cross-country ski, suspended; *muscles used:* gluteus maximus, hip flexors, core stabilizers

▶ **CUEING TIP:** Make sure the legs go backward as well as forward.

Tuck ski (see figure 2.31); *muscles used:* gluteus maximus, hip flexors, core stabilizers

▶ **CUEING TIP:** Tuck ski with a rebound or in the neutral position.

Cross-country ski, faster; *muscles used:* gluteus maximus, hip flexors

▶ **CUEING TIP:** Don't lose your range of motion.

Mini ski; *muscles used:* gluteus maximus, hip flexors

▶ **CUEING TIP:** Short and tight and fast.

Cross-country ski, full range of motion; *muscles used:* gluteus maximus, hip flexors

Cross-country ski with power; *muscles used:* gluteus maximus, hip flexors

Cross-country ski, doubles; *muscles used:* gluteus maximus, hip flexors

▶ **CUEING TIP:** Hop with the R leg forward 2×; then hop with the L leg forward 2×.

Cross-country ski, corner to corner (see figure 2.32); *muscles used:* gluteus maximus, hip flexors, obliques

▶ **CUEING TIPS:** Reach the arm across the chest. Reach across R, stop in the center, and reach across L. Increase intensity by eliminating the stop in the center.

Tuck ski, corner to corner; *muscles used:* gluteus maximus, hip flexors, core stabilizers

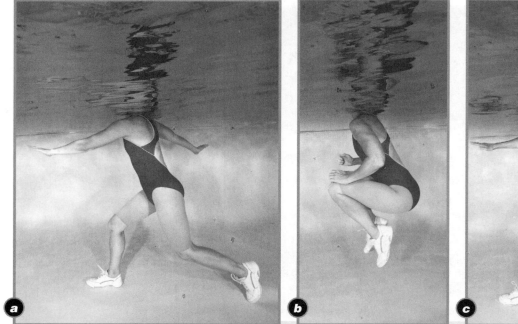
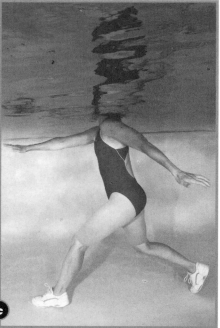

FIGURE 2.31 **Tuck ski:** *(a)* Begin in a lunge position with right leg and left arm forward; *(b)* go into a suspended tuck position; *(c)* return to a lunge position with the left leg and right arm forward.

▶ **CUEING TIP:** Reach across R, go into a suspended tuck position, and reach across L.

Cross-country ski with quarter turn; *muscles used:* gluteus maximus, hip flexors

▶ **CUEING TIP:** Ski 2–8×; then turn.

Cross-country ski 3 1/2×, half turn; *muscles used:* gluteus maximus, hip flexors

▶ **CUEING TIP:** Ski R, L, R, L, R, L, R, and turn.

Cross-country ski; travel forward, backward, or sideways

JUMPING JACKS

Jumping jacks (hip abduction and adduction; see figure 2.33); *muscles used:* gluteus medius, hip adductors

▶ **CUEING TIP:** Keep the arms underwater.

Jumping jacks with or without a bounce; *muscles used:* gluteus medius, hip adductors

Air Jordan jacks; *muscles used:* gluteus medius, hip adductors, gastrocnemius

▶ **CUEING TIP:** Use a high jump.

Jumping jacks, land with feet in only; *muscles used:* gluteus medius, hip adductors

Jumping jacks, land with feet out only; *muscles used:* gluteus medius, hip adductors

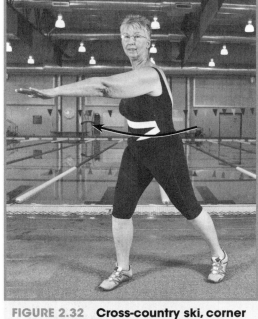

FIGURE 2.32 **Cross-country ski, corner to corner: Reach the left arm across the midline of the body as the left leg lunges toward the opposite corner.**

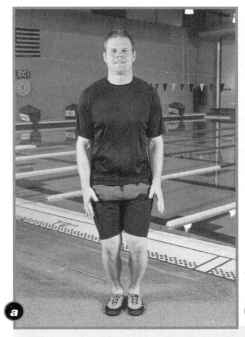
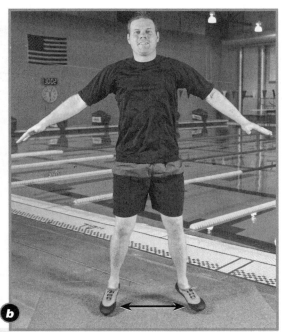

FIGURE 2.33 **Jumping jacks: *(a)* Begin with the arms down and the feet together; *(b)* abduct the shoulders as the feet come apart.**

Jumping jacks, squat; *muscles used:* gluteus medius, hip adductors, quadriceps, gluteus maximus

▶ **CUEING TIP:** Squat as the legs go apart.

Jumping jacks, neutral position; *muscles used:* tensor fasciae latae, hip adductors

Jumping jacks, suspended; suspended variations: knees bent or legs straight; *muscles used:* tensor fasciae latae, hip adductors, core stabilizers

Jacks tuck (see figure 2.34); *muscles used:* gluteus medius, core stabilizers

▶ **CUEING TIP:** Jacks tuck with a rebound or in the neutral position.

Jumping jacks, faster; *muscles used:* gluteus medius, hip adductors

▶ **CUEING TIP:** Don't lose your range of motion.

Mini jacks; *muscles used:* gluteus medius, hip adductors

▶ **CUEING TIP:** Short and tight and fast.

Mini cross; *muscles used:* gluteus medius, hip adductors

▶ **CUEING TIP:** Cross the legs in a short motion.

Triple crossover; *muscles used:* gluteus medius, hip adductors

▶ **CUEING TIP:** Mini cross 3×, jack 1×.

Jacks cross (see figure 2.35); *muscles used:* gluteus medius, hip adductors

Jacks cross, full range of motion; *muscles used:* gluteus medius, hip adductors

Jumping jacks with power; *muscles used:* gluteus medius, hip adductors

Jumping jacks, doubles; *muscles used:* gluteus medius, hip adductors

▶ **CUEING TIP:** Hop out 2×, hop in 2×.

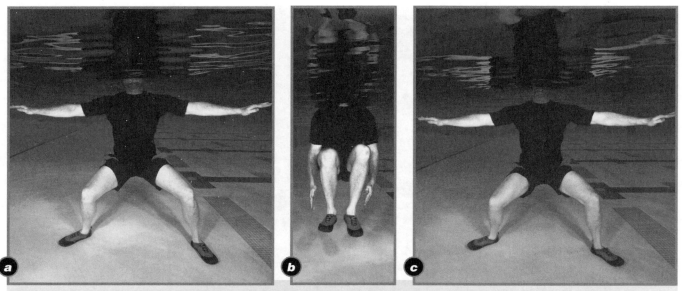

FIGURE 2.34 **Jacks tuck:** *(a)* **Begin with the shoulders abducted and the feet apart;** *(b)* **bring the arms down and go into a suspended tuck position;** *(c)* **return to the starting position.**

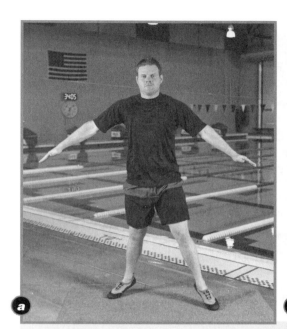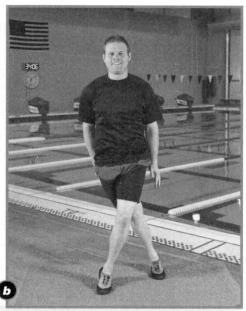

FIGURE 2.35 **Jacks cross:** *(a)* **Begin jacks cross with the feet and arms apart;** *(b)* **cross the legs as the arms come down.**

Jumping jacks with quarter turn; *muscles used:* gluteus medius, hip adductors

▶ **CUEING TIP:** Jumping jacks 2–8×; then turn.

Jacks cross 3 1/2×, half turn; *muscles used:* gluteus medius, hip adductors

▶ **CUEING TIP:** Cross, out, cross, out, cross, out, cross, and turn.

Jumping jacks; travel forward, backward, or sideways

JUMP

Jump (hip, knee, and ankle flexion and extension; see figure 2.36); *muscles used:* gastrocnemius, quadriceps, hamstrings, gluteus maximus

▶ **CUEING TIP:** Land toe-ball-heel with soft knees.

Bunny hop; *muscles used:* gastrocnemius, quadriceps, hamstrings, gluteus maximus

▶ **CUEING TIP:** Hop with the heels up.

Hop on one foot; *muscles used:* gastrocnemius, quadriceps, hamstrings, gluteus maximus, core stabilizers

Jump rope; *muscles used:* gastrocnemius, quadriceps, hamstrings, gluteus maximus

▶ **CUEING TIP:** Add arm circles as if turning the rope.

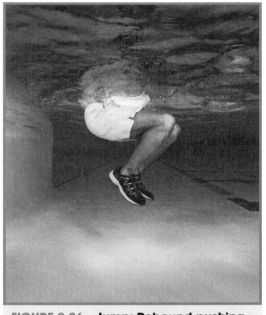

FIGURE 2.36 **Jump: Rebound pushing off the bottom of the pool with the feet.**

Squat and jump; *muscles used:* gastrocnemius, quadriceps, hamstrings, gluteus maximus

Basketball jump; *muscles used:* gastrocnemius, quadriceps, hamstrings, gluteus maximus

Jump flutter (see figure 2.37); *muscles used:* gastrocnemius, quadriceps, hamstrings, gluteus maximus, hip flexors

▶ **CUEING TIP:** Land on soft knees.

Jump backward (see figure 2.38); *muscles used:* gastrocnemius, quadriceps, core stabilizers

▶ **CUEING TIP:** Jump backward, tuck, and land.

Log jump, forward and back; *muscles used:* core stabilizers

▶ **CUEING TIP:** Log jump with a rebound or in the neutral position.

Log jump, side to side; *muscles used:* core stabilizers

▶ **CUEING TIP:** Log jump with a rebound or in the neutral position.

Jump in a circle; *muscles used:* core stabilizers

▶ **CUEING TIPS:** Jump on a clock face at 12:00, 3:00, 6:00, 9:00, and reverse. Jump in a circle with a rebound or in the neutral position.

Skateboard jump (see figure 2.39); *muscles used:* quadriceps, hamstrings, gluteus maximus

▶ **CUEING TIP:** Lunge, jump up, lunge.

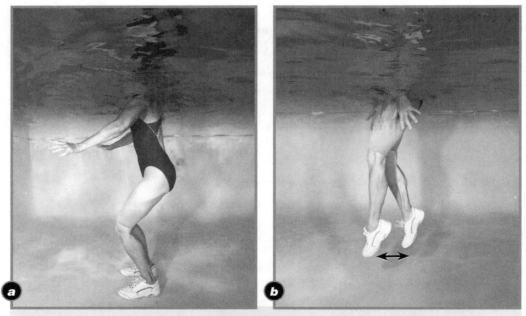

FIGURE 2.37 **Jump flutter: *(a)* Begin by bending the knees; *(b)* then jump straight up and flutter kick.**

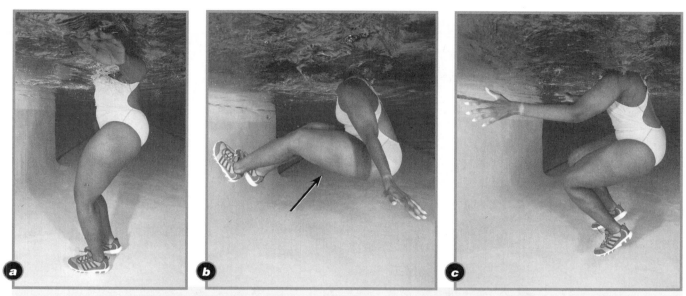

FIGURE 2.38 Jump backward: **(a)** Begin by bending the knees; **(b)** jump backward flexing at the hips; **(c)** go into a suspended tuck position and land with your feet under you.

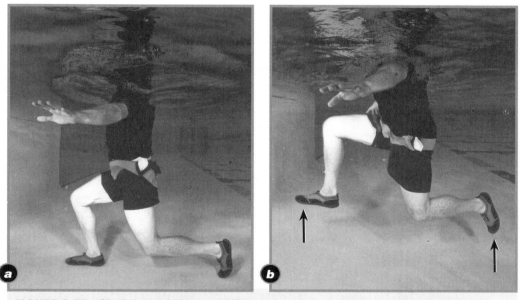

FIGURE 2.39 Skateboard jump: **(a)** Begin in a low lunge position; **(b)** jump straight up.

Frog jump (see figure 2.40); *muscles used:* gluteus medius, hip adductors

Frog jump with or without a bounce; *muscles used:* gluteus medius, hip adductors

Frog jump, neutral position; *muscles used:* gluteus medius, hip adductors

Frog jump, suspended; *muscles used:* tensor fasciae latae, hip adductors, core stabilizers

Bunny hop, jump rope, or frog jump; travel forward, backward, or sideways

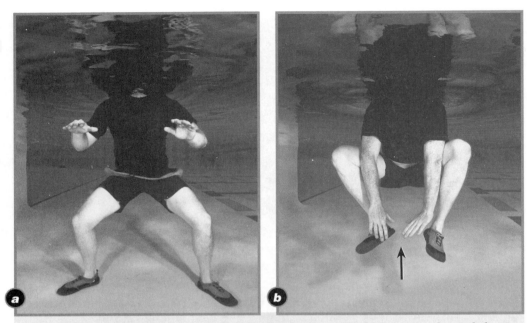

FIGURE 2.40 Frog jump: *(a)* Begin with the feet apart; *(b)* jump and reach for the ankles between the knees.

UPPER BODY

Scapula retraction; *muscles used:* trapezius, rhomboids

Crawl stroke (see figure 2.41); *muscles used:* trapezius, rhomboids

Standing row; *muscles used:* trapezius, rhomboids

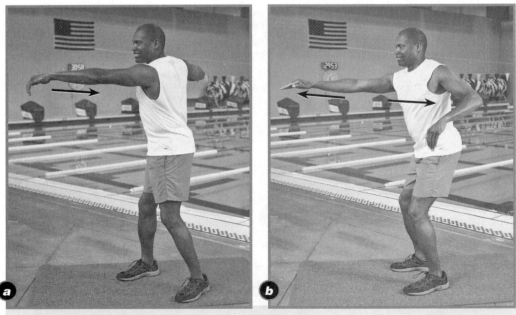

FIGURE 2.41 Crawl stroke: Reach forward and pull back with alternating arms.

Shoulder blade squeeze; *muscles used:* trapezius, rhomboids

Paddle pull; *muscles used:* trapezius, rhomboids, pectorals, obliques

▶ **CUEING TIPS:** Pull water from bellybutton to back or pull water from back to belly-button. Move the arms in unison or alternate arms.

Shoulder horizontal abduction and adduction; *muscles used:* pectorals, deltoids

Breaststroke; *muscles used:* pectorals, deltoids, trapezius, rhomboids

▶ **CUEING TIP:** Do the breaststroke with thumbs up to protect the shoulders.

Reverse breaststroke; *muscles used:* pectorals, trapezius, rhomboids

Clap hands; *muscles used:* pectorals, deltoids

Chest fly; *muscles used:* pectorals, deltoids

▶ **CUEING TIP:** Hug a barrel.

Push-ups; *muscles used:* pectorals, deltoids

▶ **CUEING TIPS:** Hold a noodle with the hands shoulder width apart and the elbows away from the body. In a lunge position push the noodle down at a 45 degree angle. For a more advanced version, do the push-ups while floating, holding the noodle below the chest. Keep the body straight, as if doing military push-ups.

Pec press, hands together; *muscles used:* pectorals

▶ **CUEING TIP:** Squeeze a volley ball.

Elbows together (see figure 2.42); *muscles used:* pectorals, deltoids

Crossovers; *muscles used:* pectorals, deltoids

▶ **CUEING TIPS:** Like clapping hands except cross arms in front. Thumbs up or palms down.

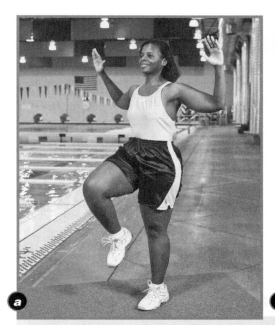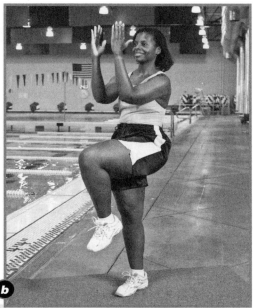

FIGURE 2.42 **Elbows together:** *(a)* **Begin with the shoulders abducted to the sides and hands up;** *(b)* **pull the elbows together in front.**

Arms sweep side to side; *muscles used:* pectorals, deltoids

Bowstring pull (see figure 2.43); *muscles used:* pectorals, deltoids, biceps

Push arm across; *muscles used:* pectorals, triceps

▶ **CUEING TIP:** Reach the arm across the chest.

Shoulder abduction and adduction; *muscles used:* latissimus dorsi, pectorals, deltoids

Lat pull-down (see figure 2.44); *muscles used:* latissimus dorsi, pectorals, deltoids

Palms touch in front; *muscles used:* pectorals, deltoids

Palms touch in back; *muscles used:* latissimus dorsi, deltoids

Arms cross in front; *muscles used:* pectorals, deltoids

Arms cross in back; *muscles used:* latissimus dorsi, deltoids

Alternate front and back; *muscles used:* latissimus dorsi, pectorals, deltoids

Lat pull-down with elbows bent; *muscles used:* latissimus dorsi, pectorals, deltoids

Arm lift to sides; *muscles used:* pectorals, deltoids

▶ **CUEING TIP:** Begin with hands crossed across chest.

Windshield wiper arms; *muscles used:* pectorals, deltoids

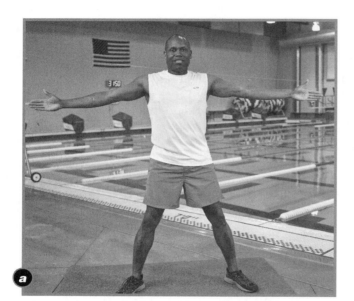
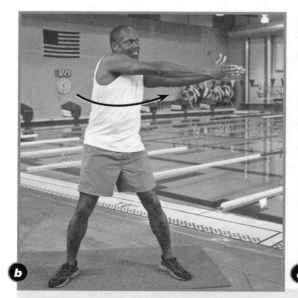
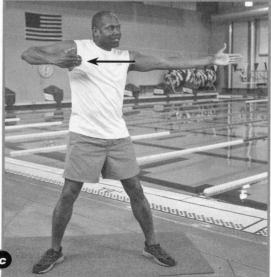

FIGURE 2.43 Bowstring pull: *(a)* Begin with the shoulders abducted to the sides; *(b)* sweep one arm across to the opposite hand; *(c)* pull the elbow back as if pulling a bowstring.

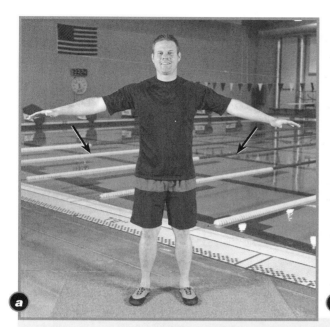
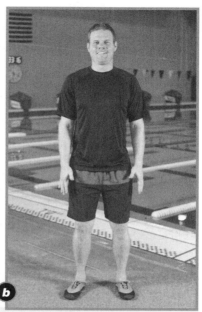

FIGURE 2.44   **Lat pull-down: *(a)* Begin with the shoulders abducted to the sides; *(b)* pull the arms down towards the body.**

Reach to the sides; *muscles used:* deltoids

Shoulder flexion and extension*; muscles used:* deltoids, latissimus dorsi

Double-arm press-down (see figure 2.45); *muscles used:* deltoids, latissimus dorsi

Double-arm lift; *muscles used:* deltoids, latissimus dorsi

Arm swing, forward and back; *muscles used:* deltoids, latissimus dorsi

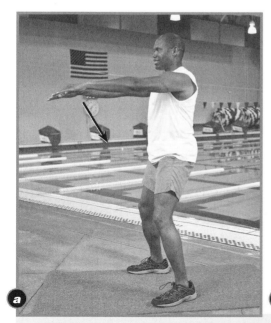
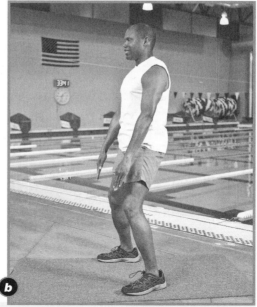

FIGURE 2.45   **Double-arm press-down: *(a)* Begin with the shoulders flexed in front; *(b)* press the arms down towards the body.**

▶ **CUEING TIPS:** Move the arms in unison or alternate arms. Increase intensity by making palms face the direction of motion.

Pumping arms; *muscles used:* deltoids, latissimus dorsi

▶ **CUEING TIP:** Pump the arms from the shoulders, not the elbows.

Shoulder lateral rotation; muscles used: rotator cuff

Forearm press (see figure 2.46); *muscles used:* rotator cuff

▶ **CUEING TIP:** Keep elbows glued to waist.

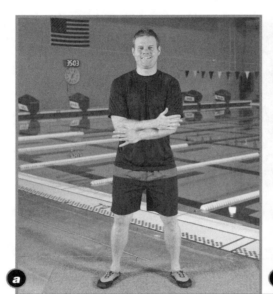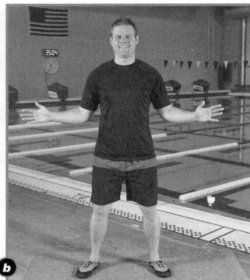

FIGURE 2.46 **Forearm press:** *(a)* **Begin with the elbows touching the waist and the hands crossed in front;** *(b)* **pull the forearms out to the sides keeping the elbows close to the waist.**

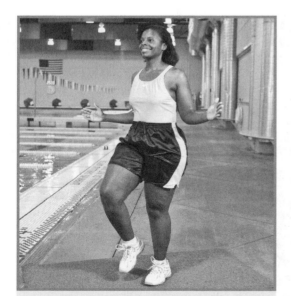

FIGURE 2.47 **Resistor arms: The elbows touch the waist and the forearms are extended to the sides.**

Forearm press, side to side; *muscles used:* rotator cuff

▶ **CUEING TIP:** Keep elbows glued to waist.

Hitchhike arms; *muscle used:* rotator cuff

Resistor arms (see figure 2.47); *muscle used:* rotator cuff

▶ **CUEING TIP:** Resistor arms add resistance when traveling forward.

Elbow flexion and extension: muscles used: biceps, triceps

Arm curl; *muscles used:* biceps, triceps

▶ **CUEING TIPS:** Move the arms in unison or alternate arms. Increase intensity by making palms face the direction of motion.

Triceps extension; *muscle used:* triceps

▶ **CUEING TIP:** Move the arms in unison or alternate arms.

Open and close doors—arm curl from shoulder abduction (see figure 2.48); *muscles used:* biceps, triceps, deltoids

Triceps press-back—triceps extension from a shoulder extension; *muscles used:* triceps, deltoids

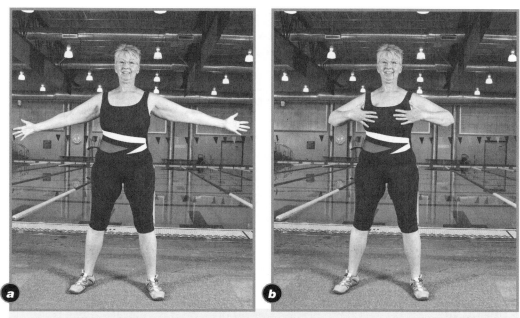

FIGURE 2.48 **Open and close doors—arm curl from shoulder abduction: *(a)*
Begin with the shoulders abducted to the sides; *(b)* flex the elbows and pull the
hands toward the chest.**

Jog press at sides or in front; *muscles used:* triceps, biceps

▶ **CUEING TIP:** Move the arms in unison or alternate arms.

Push forward (see figure 2.49); *muscle used:* triceps

▶ **CUEING TIP:** Move the arms in unison or alternate arms.

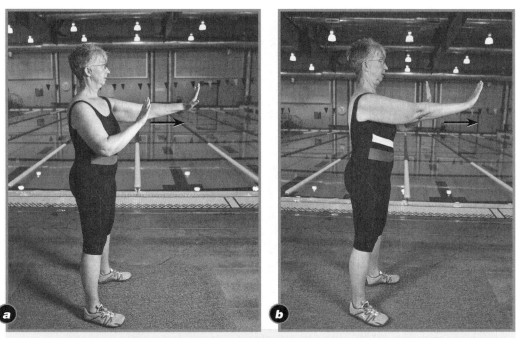

FIGURE 2.49 **Push forward: *(a)* Begin with the elbow close to the body; *(b)* push
the hand forward with the fingers up.**

Jump rope arms; *muscles used:* biceps, triceps

Paddlewheel; *muscles used:* biceps, triceps

Pronation and supination; *muscles used:* pronators, biceps

Scull; *muscles used:* pronators, biceps

▶ **CUEING TIPS:** Sweep hands out with thumbs angled down, sweep hands in with thumbs angled up. Keep the wrists locked.

Scull arms down at the sides; *muscles used:* pronators, biceps

▶ **CUEING TIP:** Make figure eights.

Wrist flexion and extension; *muscles used:* wrist flexors and extensors

Hand flutters; *muscles used:* wrist flexors and extensors

ABDOMINALS

Trunk flexion; *muscle used:* rectus abdominis

Pelvic tilt; *muscle used:* rectus abdominis

▶ **CUEING TIP:** Stand with feet hip-distance apart or sit on a noodle like a swing.

Standing crunch (see figure 2.50); *muscle used:* rectus abdominis

▶ **CUEING TIPS:** Feet hip-distance apart or lunge position. Increase intensity by holding noodle or dumbbell in hands.

Crunch, V position; *muscle used:* rectus abdominis

▶ **CUEING TIPS:** Pull the chest toward the knees. Use a noodle behind the shoulders for all suspended crunches.

Crunch with legs in a diamond position; *muscle used:* rectus abdominis

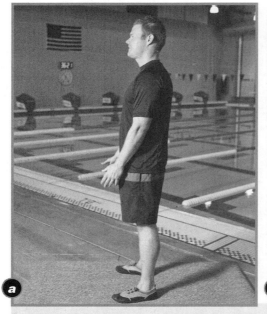 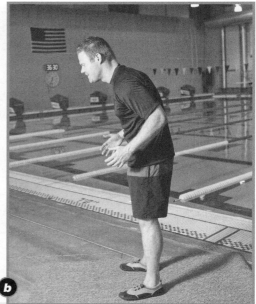

FIGURE 2.50 **Standing crunch:** *(a)* **Begin in a standing position with the spine in neutral alignment;** *(b)* **flex the trunk forward.**

Eight short crunches and two long crunches; *muscle used:* rectus abdominis

V-sit (see figure 2.51); *muscle used:* rectus abdominis

▶ **CUEING TIP:** Pull chest and straight legs together.

The hundred (Pilates); *muscle used:* rectus abdominis

▶ **CUEING TIP:** Hold V and pulse hands at sides.

Hold V and scull to travel forward; *muscle used:* rectus abdominis

Rolling like a ball (Pilates); *muscle used:* rectus abdominis

▶ **CUEING TIP:** Pull knees to chest and roll from reclining to seated with scull, noodle under knees.

Abdominal pike and spine extension (see figure 2.52); *muscles used:* rectus abdominis, erector spinae

▶ **CUEING TIPS:** Start in a seated position, extend legs forward, return to seated, and extend legs back at a 45-degree angle. Extend legs back at a 45-degree angle to avoid hyperextending the back or neck. Keep legs together. Hold a noodle in the hands. May also be done at the wall; touch feet to the wall, and then extend legs back. Advanced move is suspended with no equipment.

Abdominal pike and spine extension, legs wide in front and together in back; *muscles used:* rectus abdominis and erector spinae

Abdominal pike and spine extension, legs together in front and wide in back; *muscles used:* rectus abdominis and erector spinae

Abdominal pike and spine extension, legs wide in front and wide in back with tuck in center; *muscles used:* rectus abdominis and erector spinae

Abdominal pike and spine extension with legs in a diamond position; *muscles used:* rectus abdominis and erector spinae

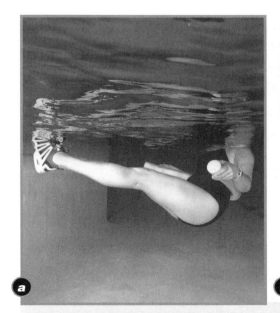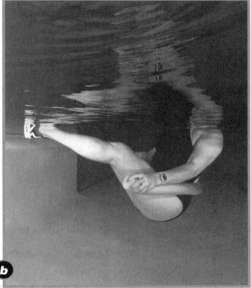

FIGURE 2.51 **V-sit:** *(a)* **Begin with the noodle behind the small of the back and the legs straight and slightly lifted;** *(b)* **pull the straight legs and the chest closer together; the hips will drop lower in the water.**

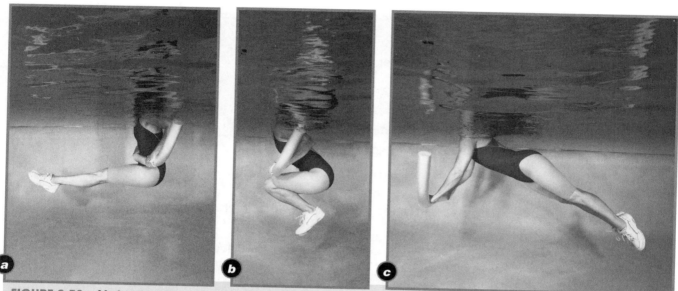

FIGURE 2.52 *Abdominal pike and spine extension: **(a)** Begin in the abdominal pike position with the noodle against the abdomen; **(b)** tuck the feet under the body; **(c)** push the noodle down in front and extend the legs to the back.*

Heels wide on floor in front, then toes on floor in center, then toes wide on floor in back; *muscles used:* core stabilizers

▶ **CUEING TIP:** Begin in the neutral position with the hips and knees flexed and the shoulders at the surface of the water. The feet are apart and the heels are on the floor. Bring the feet together under the body with the toes touching the floor. Extend the legs to the back with the feet apart and the toes touching the floor. Bring the feet under the body again with the toes touching the floor and then return to the starting position.

Hip flexion; muscles used: hip flexors; abdominals stabilize

Hip curl; *muscles used:* hip flexors, abdominals stabilize

▶ **CUEING TIPS:** Pull knees to chest. Use a noodle behind the shoulders for all hip curls.

Hip curl from a kneeling position; *muscles used:* hip flexors, abdominals stabilize

Hip curl, L position; *muscles used:* hip flexors, abdominals stabilize

Hip curl, V position; *muscles used:* hip flexors, abdominals stabilize

Hip curl with unison or alternating knees; *muscles used:* hip flexors, abdominals stabilize

Hip curl with one foot on top of the other (see figure 2.53); *muscles used:* hip flexors, abdominals stabilize

Hip curl with legs in a diamond position; *muscles used:* tensor fasciae latae, abdominals stabilize

Single-leg stretch (Pilates); *muscles used:* hip flexors, abdominals stabilize

▶ **CUEING TIP:** Begin in V position, pull one knee to chest and return to V.

Double-leg stretch (Pilates); *muscles used:* hip flexors, abdominals stabilize

▶ **CUEING TIP:** Begin in V position, pull both knees to chest and return to V.

Seated leg lift, hold for 15 seconds (see figure 2.54); *muscles used:* hip flexors, abdominals stabilize

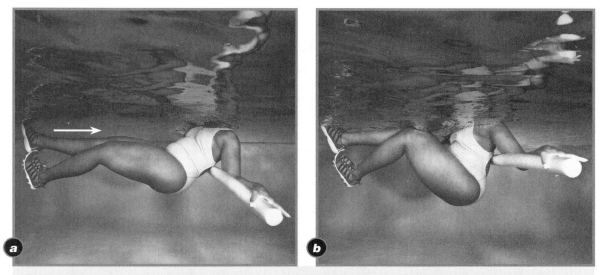

FIGURE 2.53 Hip curl with one foot on top of the other: *(a)* Begin with the noodle in the small of the back and one foot on top of the other; *(b)* flex the hips pulling the knees closer to the chest.

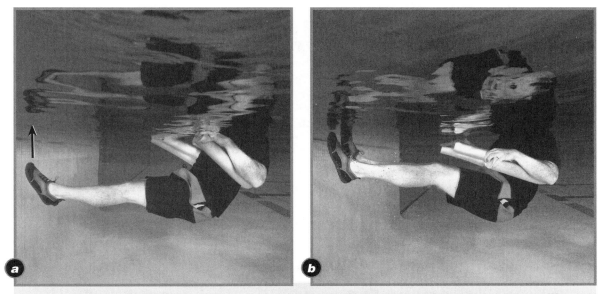

FIGURE 2.54 Seated leg lift, hold for 15 seconds: *(a)* Begin in the abdominal pike position with the noodle in the small of the back; *(b)* tighten the abdominals and flex at the hips holding the feet near the surface of the water for 15 seconds.

▶ **CUEING TIP:** Lift both legs and hold for 15 seconds.

Seated leg lift with one foot on top of the other; *muscles used:* hip flexors, abdominals stabilize

Teaser (Pilates); *muscles used:* hip flexors, abdominals stabilize

▶ **CUEING TIP:** Alternate hip curl with seated leg lift, one foot on top of the other.

OBLIQUES

Lateral rotation; muscles used: obliques

Upper-body twist (see figure 2.55); *muscles used:* obliques

Spine twist (Pilates); *muscles used:* obliques

▶ **CUEING TIP:** Perform upper-body twist slowly while straddling a noodle with legs wide apart.

Lower-body twist (see figure 2.56); *muscles used:* obliques

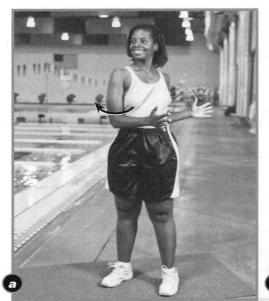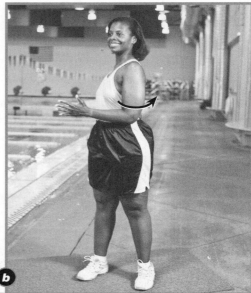

FIGURE 2.55 **Upper-body twist: Rotate the upper body from side to side.**

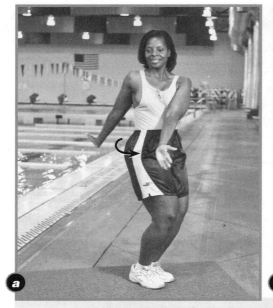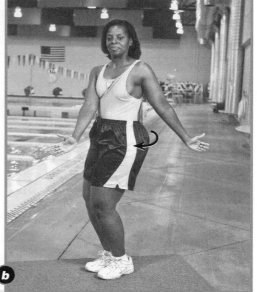

FIGURE 2.56 **Lower-body twist: Rotate the lower body from side to side.**

Hula hoop; *muscles used:* obliques

Lateral flexion; muscles used: obliques

Side crunch, standing; *muscles used:* obliques

▶ **CUEING TIPS:** Bring rib cage and pelvis closer together. Walk the fingertips down the side of one leg.

Side crunch from a kneeling position (see figure 2.57); *muscles used:* obliques

▶ **CUEING TIPS:** Bring rib cage and pelvis closer together. Use a noodle behind the shoulders for the kneeling side crunch.

Hip hike; *muscles used:* obliques

▶ **CUEING TIP:** Lift one hip at a time.

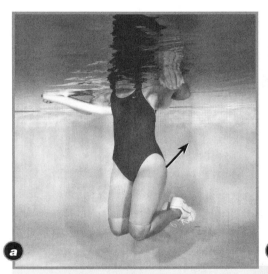 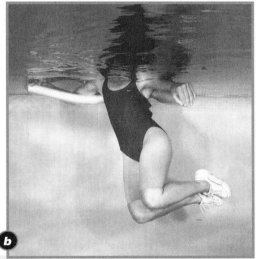

FIGURE 2.57 **Side crunch from a kneeling position: (a) Begin in a suspended kneeling position with a noodle behind the shoulders; (b) flex the trunk laterally to bring the rib cage and pelvis closer together.**

Side-lying exercises; knee high jog, side-lying; *muscles used:* obliques, hip flexors, quadriceps, hamstrings

▶ **CUEING TIP:** Use a noodle behind the shoulders or in the hands.

Bicycle, side-lying; *muscles used:* obliques, quadriceps, hamstrings

Bicycle, side-lying, in a circle; *muscles used:* obliques, quadriceps, hamstrings

Flutter kick, side-lying (see figure 2.58); *muscles used:* obliques, hip flexors, gluteus maximus

▶ **CUEING TIP:** Flutter kick from the hip.

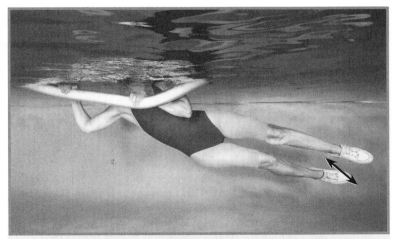

FIGURE 2.58 **Flutter kick, side-lying: Extend the legs to the side and flutter kick.**

Cross-country ski, side-lying; *muscles used:* obliques, hip flexors, gluteus maximus

Tuck ski together, side-lying (see figure 2.59); *muscles used:* obliques, hip flexors, gluteus maximus

▶ **CUEING TIP:** Tuck, ski, and pull the legs together forcefully.

Side kick (Pilates); *muscles used:* obliques, hip flexors, gluteus maximus

▶ **CUEING TIP:** In a side-lying position, move only the top leg, forward and back, slowly.

Side-to-side extension (see figure 2.60); *muscles used:* obliques

▶ **CUEING TIPS:** Extend legs to the side, tuck, and extend legs to the other side. Use a noodle behind the shoulders or in the hands. Suspended with no equipment is an advanced move.

Side-to-side extension, doubles; *muscles used:* obliques

▶ **CUEING TIP:** Extend legs to the side, tuck and extend again, and tuck and extend to the other side 2×.

Side-to-side extension with legs in a diamond position; *muscles used:* obliques

▶ **CUEING TIP:** Maintain the diamond position throughout the move.

Side-to-side extension, upper leg or lower leg only; *muscles used:* obliques

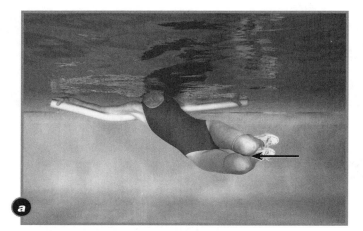

Side-to-side extension, R leg or L leg only; *muscles used:* obliques

Extension forward, R, back, L, and reverse; *muscles used:* rectus abdominis, obliques and erector spinae

▶ **CUEING TIP:** Hold a noodle in the hands.

Knee-high jog, bicycle, flutter kick, cross-country ski, or tuck ski together, side-lying; travel sideways

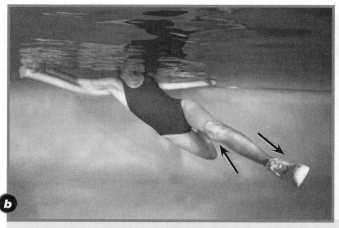

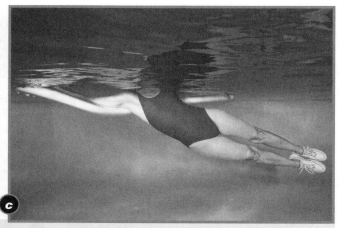

FIGURE 2.59 Tuck ski together, side-lying: *(a)* Begin in a side-lying position with the knees tucked; *(b)* take the legs apart into a cross-country ski; *(c)* pull the legs together forcefully.

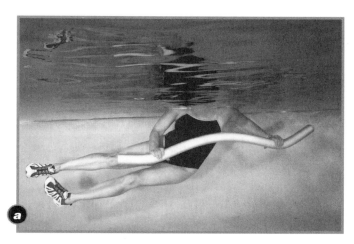

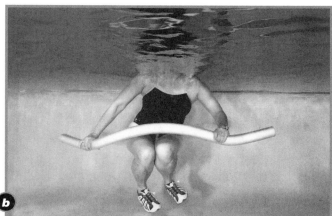

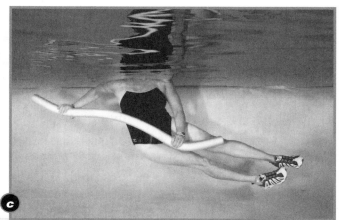

FIGURE 2.60 **Side-to-side extension: *(a)* Begin in a side-lying position; *(b)* tuck the feet under the body; *(c)* extend the legs to the opposite side.**

LOWER BODY

Bicycle (hip and knee flexion and extension; see figure 2.61); *muscles used:* hip flexors, quadriceps, hamstrings

▶ **CUEING TIP:** Use a noodle behind the shoulders, sit on it like a swing or straddle it.

Bicycle, faster; *muscles used:* hip flexors, quadriceps, hamstrings

▶ **CUEING TIP:** Don't lose your range of motion.

Bicycle, large or small circles; *muscles used:* hip flexors, quadriceps, hamstrings

Bicycle, climb a hill; *muscles used:* hip flexors, quadriceps, hamstrings

▶ **CUEING TIPS:** Put your bicycle in first gear and climb a hill. Use power.

Bicycle, one leg only; *muscles used:* hip flexors, quadriceps, hamstrings, core stabilizers

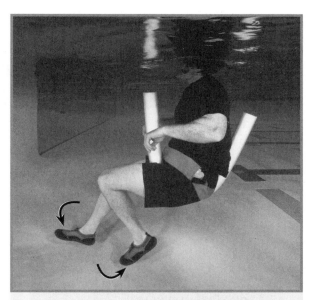

FIGURE 2.61 **Bicycle: Pedal the feet in a circular motion.**

Bicycle, tandem; *muscles used:* hip flexors, quadriceps, hamstrings, core stabilizers

▶ **CUEING TIP:** Bicycle with legs in unison.

Bicycle, reverse; *muscles used:* hip flexors, quadriceps, hamstrings

Bicycle, travel forward or backward

Seated leg press (hip and knee extension; see figure 2.62); *muscles used:* quadriceps, gluteus maximus

▶ **CUEING TIPS:** Use a noodle behind the shoulders or straddle it. Push heels forward; point toes slightly out.

Seated kick (knee flexion and extension; see figure 2.63); *muscles used:* quadriceps, hamstrings

▶ **CUEING TIPS:** Use a noodle behind the shoulders, sit on it like a swing or straddle it. Keep knees soft. Participants with knee problems may wish to substitute a seated leg press for the seated kick.

Seated kick, feet pointed or flexed; *muscles used:* quadriceps, hamstrings

Mermaid—unison kick (see figure 2.64); *muscles used:* quadriceps, hamstrings, core stabilizers

▶ **CUEING TIP:** Like pumping a swing.

Seated flutter kick (hip flexion); *muscles used:* hip flexors

▶ **CUEING TIPS:** Use a noodle behind the shoulders or sit on it like a swing. Flutter kick from the hip, not the knees. Floppy feet.

Flutter kick up to L position and down to the floor (see figure 2.65); *muscles used:* hip flexors, core stabilizers

Seated high kick (hip flexion and extension; see figure 2.66); *muscles used:* gluteus maximus, hip flexors

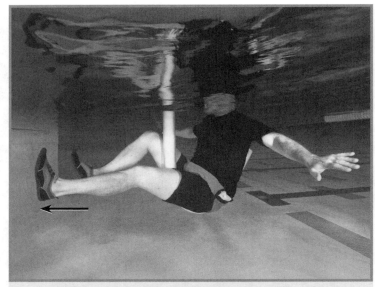

FIGURE 2.62 Seated leg press: Push the heels forward one foot at a time.

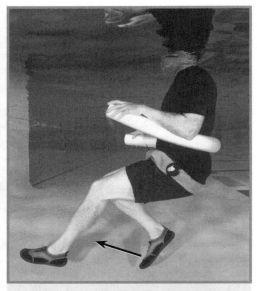

FIGURE 2.63 Seated kick: Kick from the knees in a seated position.

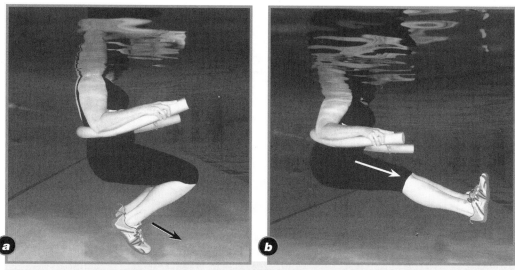

FIGURE 2.64 Mermaid—unison kick: *(a)* Begin by flexing the knees and pulling the heels under the body; *(b)* extend the knees.

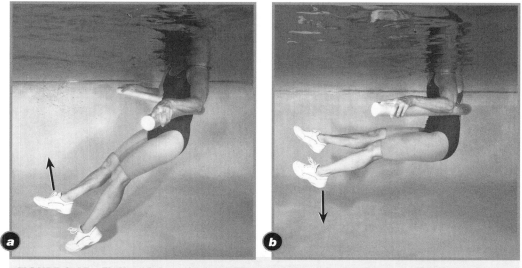

FIGURE 2.65 Flutter kick up to L position and down to the floor: *(a)* Begin the flutter kick with the feet near the floor; *(b)* walk the flutter kick up to the L position.

▶ **CUEING TIPS:** Use a noodle behind the shoulders. Emphasize the down action.

Seated Cossack kick (hip abduction and knee flexion and extension; see figure 2.67); *muscles used:* gluteus medius, quadriceps, hamstrings

▶ **CUEING TIPS:** Use a noodle behind the shoulders. Sit with legs in a diamond position and kick to the sides.

Seated jacks (horizontal hip abduction and adduction; see figure 2.68); *muscles used:* tensor fasciae latae, hip adductors

▶ **CUEING TIP:** Use a noodle behind the shoulders or straddle it.

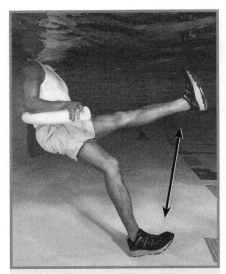

FIGURE 2.66 Seated high kick: Kick from the hips bringing the toes to the surface of the water and the heels to the floor.

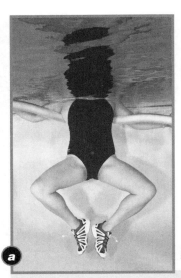

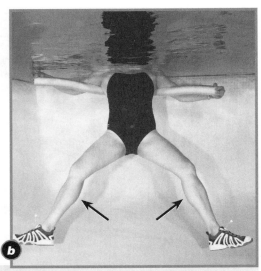

FIGURE 2.67 Seated Cossack kick: (a) Begin in a seated position with hips abducted and the heels together; **(b)** kick from the knees out to the sides.

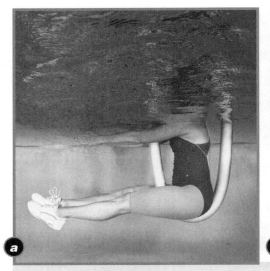

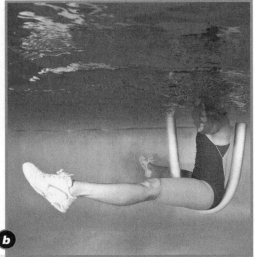

FIGURE 2.68 Seated jacks: (a) Straddle a noodle with the hips and shoulders flexed; **(b)** abduct the arms and legs horizontally.

Seated jacks, toes in or out; *muscles used:* tensor fasciae latae, hip adductors

Seated jacks cross; *muscles used:* tensor fasciae latae, hip adductors

Seated mini cross; *muscles used:* tensor fasciae latae, hip adductors

Seated triple crossover; *muscles used:* tensor fasciae latae, hip adductors

▶ **CUEING TIP:** Mini cross 3×, jack 1×.

Seated breaststroke (see figure 2.69) *and reverse breaststroke* (horizontal hip abduction and adduction); *muscles used:* tensor fasciae latae, hip adductors

▶ **CUEING TIPS:** Straddle a noodle. Arms and legs do the same thing.

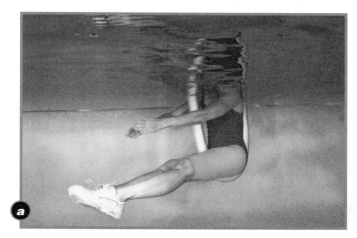

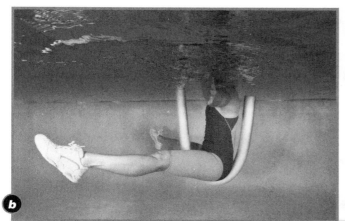

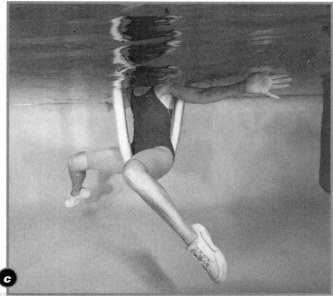

FIGURE 2.69 **Seated breaststroke: (a) Begin with the hips and shoulders flexed; (b) abduct the arms and legs horizontally in a breaststroke motion; (c) flex the elbows and knees to return to the starting position.**

Hip extension; muscle used: gluteus maximus

Rock climb (see figure 2.70); *muscle used:* gluteus maximus

▶ **CUEING TIP:** Noodle under chest; feet don't touch the floor.

Knee lift, straighten leg and power-press down; *muscle used:* gluteus maximus

BALANCE

Walk forward with arms folded, legs straight; *muscles used:* core stabilizers

Walk forward, hands up; *muscles used:* core stabilizers

Knee-high jog, pause on one foot with posture check; *muscles used:* core stabilizers

Walk forward three steps and stand on one foot with posture check; *muscles used:* core stabilizers

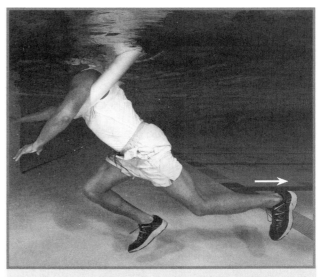

FIGURE 2.70 **Rock climb: Lean forward on a noodle and perform a climbing motion pressing the heels back.**

Stand on one foot and extend leg, hands up; *muscles used:* core stabilizers

Fall forward, tuck and stand (see figure 2.71); *muscles used:* core stabilizers

▶ **CUEING TIP:** May be done with noodle or dumbbells or no equipment.

Fall forward, tuck and stand on one foot; *muscles used:* core stabilizers

Diamond fall forward, tuck and stand; *muscles used:* core stabilizers

▶ **CUEING TIP:** Fall forward with legs in a diamond position, hips open and heels together.

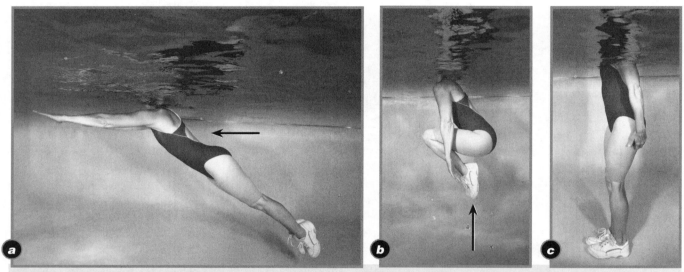

FIGURE 2.71 **Fall forward, tuck and stand:** *(a)* **Begin by falling forward keeping the arms near the surface of the water;** *(b)* **go into a suspended tuck position;** *(c)* **land with your feet under you.**

Side fall, tuck and stand (see figure 2.72); *muscles used:* core stabilizers, obliques

▶ **CUEING TIP:** May be done with noodle or dumbbells or no equipment.

Side fall, tuck and stand on one foot; *muscles used:* core stabilizers, obliques

Heels out, then toes in (see figure 2.73); *muscles used:* core stabilizers

▶ **CUEING TIPS:** Begin in the neutral position with the hips and knees flexed and the shoulders at the surface of the water. The feet are apart and the heels are on the floor. Bring the feet together under the body with the toes touching the floor and then return to the starting position.

Heels out, then chair position suspended; *muscles used:* core stabilizers

▶ **CUEING TIPS:** Begin in the neutral position with the hips and knees flexed and the shoulders at the surface of the water. The feet are apart and the heels are on the floor. Bring the feet together under the body in a suspended tuck position.

Heels out, then chair position suspended, then L position, then chair position suspended (see figure 2.74); *muscles used:* core stabilizers

▶ **CUEING TIPS:** Begin in the neutral position with the hips and knees flexed and the shoulders at the surface of the water. The feet are apart and the heels are on the floor. Bring the feet together under the body in a suspended tuck position. Straighten the legs in an abdominal pike then return to the suspended tuck position.

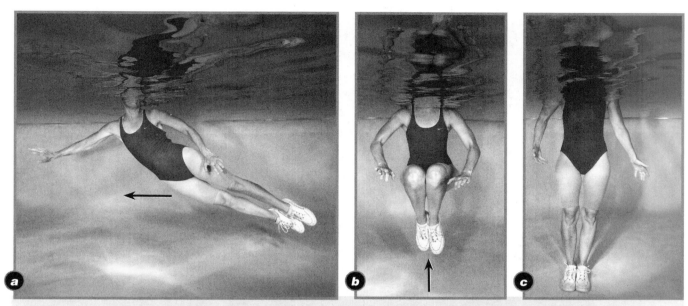

FIGURE 2.72 Side fall, tuck and stand: *(a)* Begin by falling sideways keeping the arm near the surface of the water; *(b)* go into a suspended tuck position; *(c)* land with your feet under you.

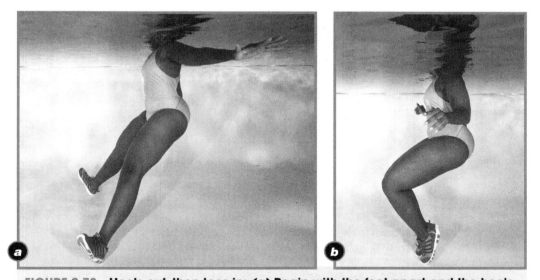

FIGURE 2.73 Heels out, then toes in: *(a)* Begin with the feet apart and the heels on the floor; *(b)* bring the feet together under the body with the toes touching the floor.

Standing leg press with one foot on noodle; *muscles used:* core stabilizers, quadriceps, gluteus maximus

Cross-country ski with one foot on noodle; *muscles used:* core stabilizers

Jumping jacks with one foot on noodle; *muscles used:* core stabilizers

Kneel on noodle and balance; *muscles used:* core stabilizers

Kneel on noodle; travel with breaststroke, reverse breaststroke, or sidestroke; *muscles used:* core stabilizers

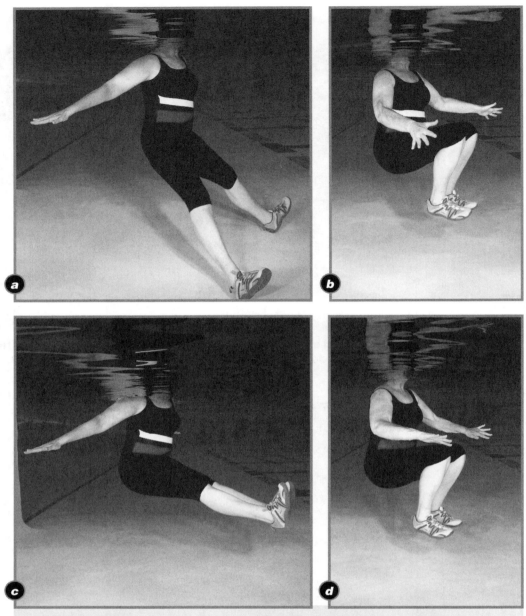

FIGURE 2.74 Heels out, then chair position suspended, then L position, then chair position suspended: *(a)* Begin with the feet apart and the heels on the floor; *(b)* bring the feet together under the body in a suspended tuck position; *(c)* straighten the legs in an abdominal pike; *(d)* return to the suspended tuck position.

Stand on noodle and use as a stair climber; *muscles used:* core stabilizers, quadriceps, gluteus maximus

▶ **CUEING TIP:** Lift one knee at a time and press the noodle down to the floor.

Stand on noodle and balance with one leg lifted forward (see figure 2.75); *muscles used:* core stabilizers

Stand on noodle and balance with one leg extended backward; *muscles used:* core stabilizers

Stand on noodle and hop in place or travel; *muscles used:* core stabilizers

Hop with one leg lifted forward or extended backward; *muscles used:* core stabilizers

Surf (see figure 2.76); *muscles used:* core stabilizers

▶ **CUEING TIP:** Stand on noodle and pull knees to chest; noodle comes off the floor.

Surf; travel with breaststroke, reverse breaststroke, or sidestroke; *muscles used:* core stabilizers

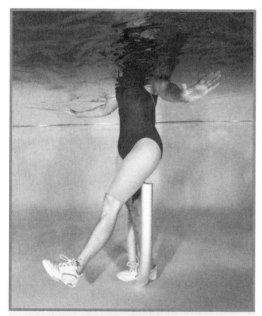

FIGURE 2.75 Stand on noodle and balance with one leg lifted forward: One foot is on the noodle and the other leg is lifted forward.

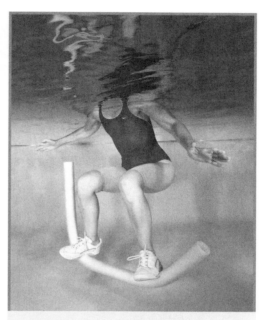

FIGURE 2.76 Surf: Both feet are on the noodle hip distance apart; float with the hips and knees flexed.

CHAPTER 3

Shallow-Water Lesson Plans

Choreography is the way you organize your lesson plan to give it logic and flow and make it easy to remember. This book presents four strategies for developing choreography. They are linear choreography, variations on a theme, add-on choreography, and block choreography.

LINEAR CHOREOGRAPHY

Linear choreography is an easy way to organize a lesson plan. You simply write a list of exercises without repetition, or with very little repetition. Linear choreography can be represented by letters (a, b, c, d, e). Begin with exercise "a" and then go to exercise "b" and so on until you have enough material to fill up your class time. Be sure to include a warm-up, a conditioning phase, and a cool-down. It is helpful to have some kind of theme to your linear choreography so it doesn't feel like just a random list of exercises. Your theme might be an introduction to basic moves, strength training, a circuit class, shallow-water running, traveling, or using noodles.

▶ **Shallow-Water Lesson Plan 1**

BASIC MOVES

CLASS OBJECTIVE
Cardiorespiratory fitness

EQUIPMENT
Noodles

TEACHING TIP
This class introduces basic moves to new participants, but it also provides experienced participants with a cardiorespiratory workout. Be sure to cue good posture—*ears over shoulders, shoulders over hips, feet under you.* For the arm medley, choose any upper-body moves you like.

WARM-UP
Knee-high jog

Crossover knees

Run tires

In in, out out

Run tires, travel backward and forward

Run tires, travel sideways

CONDITIONING PHASE
(A set)

Knee-high jog with arm medley

Sprint

Heel jog, push forward, travel backward and forward

Skateboard

Rocking horse

Cross-country ski

Tuck ski

Cross-country ski, suspended

Cross-country ski, travel backward and forward

Cross-country ski, travel sideways

(B set)

Kick forward with breaststroke, travel backward and forward

High kick, travel backward and forward

Jump backward

Leap forward (low-impact option: sprint)

Kick side to side, travel sideways

Jumping jacks, travel sideways

Jumping jacks, clap hands, travel backward and forward

Jacks cross

Jumping jacks, squat

(C set)

Ankle touch

Hopscotch

In-line skate

Skate kick with pumping arms, travel backward and forward

Skip rope

Hop on one foot (low-impact option: walk on heels)

Crab walk sideways

COOL-DOWN
(Noodle behind shoulders)

Flutter kick, side-lying

Bicycle, side-lying, in a circle

Bicycle

Seated kick, feet pointed

Seated kick, feet flexed

Seated flutter kick

Seated pelvic tilt

Standing crunch

Fall forward, tuck and stand

Side fall, tuck and stand

Stretch: hip flexors, quadriceps, gastrocnemius, hamstrings, lower back, shoulders

▶ **Shallow-Water Lesson Plan 2**

ARM MOVES, CHANGE LEGS

CLASS OBJECTIVE
Muscular strength and endurance

EQUIPMENT
Noodles

TEACHING TIP
Have participants do three sets of 16 repetitions with each upper-body move, but use a different leg move with each set. Have them shake their arms out and rest them between sets, continuing the leg move without using the arms for eight repetitions. When

they change to the next leg move, they should resume the arm moves.

WARM-UP

Instructor's choice

CONDITIONING PHASE

(A set)
Shoulder blade squeeze with knee-high jog
Shoulder blade squeeze with rocking horse
Shoulder blade squeeze with heel jog
Sprint

(B set)
Clap hands with knee-high jog
Clap hands with jumping jacks
Clap hands with jacks cross
Sprint

(C set)
Pec press, hands together, with knee-high jog
Pec press, hands together, with kick forward
Pec press, hands together, with skate kick
Sprint

(D set)
Arm swing with knee-high jog
Arm swing with kick forward
Arm swing with cross-country ski
Sprint

(E set)
Lat pull-down with knee-high jog
Lat pull-down with jumping jacks
Lat pull-down with high kick
Sprint

(F set)
Arm curl with knee-high jog
Arm curl with rocking horse
Arm curl with run tires
Sprint

(G set)
Triceps extension with knee-high jog
Triceps extension with kick side to side
Triceps extension with run tires
Sprint

(H set)
Forearm press with knee-high jog
Forearm press with cross-country ski
Forearm press with heel jog
Knee-high jog, travel forward

COOL-DOWN

(Noodle behind shoulders)
Flutter kick up to L position and down to the floor
Flutter kick, side-lying
Side-to-side extension
Hip curl with one foot on top of the other
Seated leg lift with one foot on top of the other
Teaser (Pilates)
Stretch: upper back, pectorals, shoulders, latissimus dorsi, triceps, gastrocnemius

▶ **Shallow-Water Lesson Plan 3**

LEG MOVES, CHANGE ARMS 1

CLASS OBJECTIVES

Cardiorespiratory fitness and muscular strength and endurance

EQUIPMENT

None

TEACHING TIP

If participants keep their legs moving while they perform 8 to 12 repetitions of each strength training exercise for the upper body, their heart rates will stay in the lower level of their target heart rates. Adding travel on every third strength training exercise will increase not only the resistance for the upper body but also the heart rate. If you add four sets of intervals to bring them into the upper level of their target heart rates, you will accomplish two objectives in one class. In the lesson plans in this book, the exercises used to bring the heart rate up during interval sessions are labeled *interval high intensity phase*. The exercises used to decrease heart rate following the high-intensity phase are labeled *interval active recovery phase*.

WARM-UP

Instructor's choice

CONDITIONING PHASE

(A set)
Knee-high jog with jog press

Knee-high jog with crossovers, emphasize pectorals

Knee-high jog with unison push forward, travel backward and forward

Interval high-intensity phase: knee-high jog, faster

Interval active recovery phase: knee-high jog

(B set)

Run tires, reach to the sides

Run tires with crossovers, emphasize posterior deltoids

Run tires with double-arm press-down, travel backward and forward

(C set)

Cross-country ski, push forward

Cross-country ski with forearm press, side to side

Cross-country ski with unison arm swing, travel backward and forward

Interval high-intensity phase: cross-country ski with power

Interval active recovery phase: cross-country ski

(D set)

Jumping jacks, arms cross in back

Jumping jacks with lat pull-down with elbows bent

Jumping jacks, clap hands, travel backward and forward

(E set)

Kick forward with triceps press-back

Kick forward with arm lift to sides

Kick forward with crawl stroke, travel backward and forward

Interval high-intensity phase: kick forward, faster

Interval active recovery phase: kick forward

(F set)

Kick side to side with windshield wiper arms

Kick side to side, arms sweep side to side

Kick side to side, arms cross in front, travel backward and forward

(G set)

Heel jog, scull arms down

Heel jog with standing row

Heel jog with hand flutters, travel backward and forward

Interval high-intensity phase: skateboard, faster

Interval active recovery phase: skateboard

(H set)

Rocking horse with shoulder blade squeeze

Rocking horse with forearm press

Rocking horse with arm curl, travel backward and forward

COOL-DOWN

Walk forward, hands up

Walk forward three steps and stand on one foot with posture check

Standing pelvic tilt

Upper-body twist

Hip hike

Crunch, lunge position

Stretch: upper back, pectorals, shoulders, latissimus dorsi, triceps, hip flexors

▶ Shallow-Water Lesson Plan 4

LEG MOVES, CHANGE ARMS 2

CLASS OBJECTIVES

Cardiorespiratory fitness and muscular strength and endurance

EQUIPMENT

Noodles

TEACHING TIP

Have participants keep their legs moving while they perform 8 to 12 repetitions of each strength training exercise for the upper body. After three sets of strength training exercises, they do a set of intervals to bring them into the upper level of their target heart rates.

WARM-UP

Instructor's choice

CONDITIONING PHASE

(A set)

Cross-country ski

Cross-country ski with unison arm swing

Cross-country ski with windshield wiper arms

Interval high-intensity phase: cross-country ski, neutral position, full ROM

Interval active recovery phase: cross-country ski, neutral position

(B set)

Jumping jacks

Jumping jacks, palms touch in front and in back

Jumping jacks, clap hands

Interval high-intensity phase: mini jacks, faster

Interval active recovery phase: jumping jacks

(C set)

Kick forward with arm swing, palms face direction of motion

Kick forward, elbows together

Kick forward with jump rope arms

Interval high-intensity phase: high kick

Interval active recovery phase: kick forward

(D set)

Kick side to side

Kick side to side with hitchhike arms

Kick side to side with bowstring pull

Interval high-intensity phase: kick side to side, arms and legs opposite, with power

Interval active recovery phase: kick side to side

(E set)

Skate kick with pumping arms

Skate kick, push arm across

Skate kick with paddlewheel

Interval high-intensity phase: kick and lunge

Interval active recovery phase: skate kick

(F set)

Heel jog with chest fly

Heel jog with breaststroke

Heel jog, open and close doors

Interval high-intensity phase: kick forward, suspended, emphasize hamstrings

Interval active recovery phase: kick forward, neutral position

(G set)

Knee-high jog with standing row

Knee-high jog with reverse breaststroke

Knee-high jog with triceps extension

Interval high-intensity phase: steep climb

Interval active recovery phase: knee-high jog

COOL-DOWN

(Noodle behind shoulders)

Hip curl from a kneeling position

Side crunch from a kneeling position

Crunch, V position

Side-to-side extension

Side-to-side extension, upper leg only

Side-to-side extension, lower leg only

Stretch: upper back, pectorals, shoulders, latissimus dorsi, triceps, gastrocnemius

▶ Shallow-Water Lesson Plan 5

CIRCUIT WORKOUT 1

CLASS OBJECTIVE

Muscular strength and endurance

EQUIPMENT

Noodles (dumbbells are optional)

TEACHING TIP

At the end of each set of rhythmic exercises, have participants stabilize their bodies in a lunge or squat position before performing the upper-body strength training exercises with dumbbells or hands cupped. Remind them to push hard against the resistance of the water. The last exercise before stretching is rolling like a ball. If you have participants who feel uncomfortable reclining with a noodle under the knees, then you may want to skip this exercise.

WARM-UP

Instructor's choice

CONDITIONING PHASE

(A set)

Knee-high jog, travel backward and forward

Heel jog, travel backward and forward

Rocking horse, travel backward and forward

Run tires, travel sideways

Palms touch in front (lunge position)

Palms touch in back (lunge position)

(B set)

Jumping jacks; travel backward, forward, and sideways

Jacks tuck

Jumping jacks, suspended

Crossovers, emphasize posterior deltoids (lunge position)

Crossovers, emphasize pectorals (lunge position)

(C set)

Kick forward, travel backward and forward

Kick forward, neutral position, travel backward and forward

Small kick

High kick

Breaststroke (lunge position)

Reverse breaststroke (lunge position)

(D set)

Cross-country ski; travel backward, forward, and sideways

Tuck ski

Cross-country ski, suspended

Shoulder blade squeeze (lunge position)

Standing row (lunge position)

(E set)

Crossover knees

Crossover kick

Chorus line kick

Jump flutter (low-impact option: skip rope)

Double-arm press-down (squat position)

Push arm across (squat position)

(F set)

Skate kick

One leg kicks forward and back

Log jump, forward and back

Jump backward and leap forward (low-impact option: jump backward and sprint forward)

Arm curl (lunge position)

Open and close doors (squat position)

(G set)

Kick side to side

Side kick (karate)

Log jump, side to side

Walk forward with arms folded, legs straight

Triceps extension (squat position)

Push forward (squat position)

COOL-DOWN

(Sit on noodle)

Pelvic tilt

(Noodle behind shoulders)

Hip curl, L position

Hip curl with alternating knees

The hundred (Pilates)

(Noodle under knees)

Rolling like a ball (Pilates)

Stretch: upper back, pectorals, shoulders, latissimus dorsi, triceps, quadriceps

▶ Shallow-Water Lesson Plan 6

CIRCUIT WORKOUT 2

CLASS OBJECTIVE

Muscular strength and endurance

EQUIPMENT

None

TEACHING TIP

This lesson plan focuses on the muscles on the back of the body, which are used less often than the muscles in front. Traveling backward increases the resistance.

WARM-UP

Knee-high jog with jog press

Straddle jog with shoulder blade squeeze

Knee-high jog, palms touch in back

Knee-high jog with scull

Knee-high jog, faster, with scull

Knee-high jog, scull arms down, travel forward

CONDITIONING PHASE

(A set)

Knee-high jog with breaststroke, travel backward

Knee-high jog with shoulder blade squeeze, travel backward

Knee-high jog with standing row, travel backward

Knee-high jog, palms touch in back, travel backward

Knee-high jog, travel backward; sprint, travel in a zigzag

(B set)

High kick, travel backward and forward

Skate kick, travel backward and forward

Cross-country ski, travel backward and forward

Knee lift and lunge

Knee-high jog, travel in a square and change directions

(C set)

Knee-high jog with triceps press-back, travel backward

Knee-high jog with triceps extension, travel backward

Knee-high jog, push forward, travel backward and forward

Knee-high jog with unison jog press, travel backward and forward

Knee-high jog with quick change of direction

(D set)

Rocking horse, travel backward

Heel jog, travel backward

Cossack kick, neutral position

Kick forward, suspended, emphasize hamstrings

Knee-high jog, travel in a circle and reverse

(E set)

Jumping jacks, travel sideways

Jumping jacks, emphasize adduction

Jacks cross

Kick side to side, arms and legs opposite

One leg kicks side

Knee-high jog, travel backward; sprint, travel in a zigzag

Knee-high jog, travel in a square and change directions

Knee-high jog with quick change of direction

Knee-high jog, travel in a circle and reverse

COOL-DOWN

Fall forward, tuck and stand on one foot

Side fall, tuck and stand on one foot

Crunch, lunge position

Heels out, then chair position suspended

Heels out, then chair position suspended, then L position, then chair position suspended

Mermaid, suspended

Stretch: upper back, lower back, triceps, hamstrings, inner thigh, neck

▶ Shallow-Water Lesson Plan 7

CIRCUIT WORKOUT 3

CLASS OBJECTIVE

Muscular strength and endurance

EQUIPMENT

Noodles

TEACHING TIP

Have participants travel for four minutes and then do a strength training exercise for one minute to improve muscular endurance. This lesson plan focuses on the muscles on the back of the body, which are used less often than the muscles in front. The targeted muscles are listed in parentheses after each strength training exercise.

WARM-UP

Knee-high jog

Straddle jog

Kick side to side

Ankle touch

Hopscotch

Jumping jacks

Jacks tuck

Tuck ski

Cross-country ski

CONDITIONING PHASE

(A set)

Sprint, hands fisted (1 min.)

Sprint, hands cupped (1 min.)

Repeat both

Knee-high jog with crossovers, travel backward (posterior deltoids) (1 min.)

(B set)

Knee-high jog with breaststroke, travel forward (1 min.)

Knee-high jog with reverse breaststroke, travel backward (1 min.)

Repeat both

Knee lift, straighten leg and power-press down, travel backward (gluteus maximus) (1 min.)

(C set)

Knee-high jog with double-arm press-down, travel forward (1 min.)

Knee-high jog, scull in front, travel backward (1 min.)

Repeat both

Knee-high jog with triceps extension, travel backward (triceps) (1 min.)

(D set)

Knee-high jog with crawl stroke, travel forward (1 min.)

Knee-high jog, push forward, travel backward (1 min.)

Repeat both

Skateboard jump (hamstrings) (30 secs.)

(E set)

Sprint with resistor arms (1 min.)

Sprint with breaststroke (1 min.)

Repeat both

Lat pull-down, lunge position (latissimus dorsi) (1 min.)

(F set)

Sprint, hands cupped (1 min.)

Knee-high jog, hands fisted, travel forward (1 min.)

Repeat both

One leg kicks side (gluteus medius and adductors) (30 secs. each side)

COOL-DOWN

(Noodle in hands)

Abdominal pike and spine extension

Side-to-side extension

(Noodle under chest)

Rock climb

(Stand on noodle)

Balance with one leg lifted forward

Balance with one leg extended backward

Stretch: upper back, lower back, triceps, hamstrings, latissimus dorsi, shoulders

▶ Shallow-Water Lesson Plan 8

SINGLES AND DOUBLES

CLASS OBJECTIVE

Cardiorespiratory fitness

EQUIPMENT

Noodles

TEACHING TIP

Single, single, double moves are a fun way to challenge coordination. For these moves, participants will perform the exercise with the right leg 1×, the left leg 1× and the right leg 2×, then with the left leg 1×, the right leg 1× and the left leg 2×, and so on.

WARM-UP

Instructor's choice

CONDITIONING PHASE

(A set)

Knee-high jog

Knee-high jog, doubles

Knee-high jog, single, single, double

Jump rope (low impact option: skip rope)

Run tires

Run tires, doubles

Run tires, single, single, double

Frog jump (low-impact option: neutral position)

Heel jog

Heel jog, doubles

Heel jog, single, single, double

Bunny hop (low-impact option: skateboard)

High kick, travel backward and forward

Jumping jacks, clap hands, travel backward and forward

(B set)

Ankle touch

Ankle touch, doubles

Ankle touch, single, single, double

Hopscotch

Hopscotch, doubles

Hopscotch, single, single, double

High kick, travel backward and forward

Jumping jacks, clap hands, travel backward and forward

(C set)

Knee-high jog, push forward and unison push forward

Knee-high jog with jog press in front and unison jog press in front

Knee-high jog with jog press at sides and unison jog press at sides

Knee-high jog with alternating arm curl and unison arm curl

Cross-country ski with arm swing and unison arm swing

Cross-country ski with forearm press and forearm press, side to side

Leap forward (low-impact option: lunge forward low in the water)

Leap sideways (low-impact option: squat travel sideways)

(D set)

Kick forward

Kick forward, doubles

Kick forward, single, single, double

Jump backward

Jumping jacks

Jumping jacks, doubles

Jumping jacks, single, single, double

Cross-country ski, travel forward

Cross-country ski

Cross-country ski, doubles

Cross-country ski, single, single, double

Tuck ski

Tuck ski, doubles

Tuck ski, single, single, double

Kick forward, travel backward and forward

Jumping jacks, travel backward and forward

COOL-DOWN

(Noodle behind shoulders)

Seated kick

Mermaid

Hip curl with alternating knees

Hip curl with unison knees

Seated leg lift, hold for 15 seconds

Side-to-side extension

Side-to-side extension, doubles

Stretch: quadriceps, hamstrings, gastrocnemius, inner thigh, shoulders, upper back

▶ Shallow-Water Lesson Plan 9

CORE CHALLENGE

CLASS OBJECTIVE

Core strength

EQUIPMENT

Noodles

TEACHING TIP

Good core strength helps maintain good posture.

WARM-UP

Instructor's choice

CONDITIONING PHASE

(A set)

High kick, travel backward and forward

Jumping jacks, travel sideways

Skate kick, travel backward and forward

High kick

R leg kicks forward 12×, L leg kicks forward 12×

Jumping jacks

R leg kicks side 12×, L leg kicks side 12×

Skate kick with pumping arms

R leg kicks back 12×, L leg kicks back 12×

High kick, travel backward and forward

Jumping jacks, travel sideways

Skate kick, travel backward and forward

High kick

R leg kicks forward and side 8×, L leg kicks forward and side 8×

Jumping jacks

R leg kicks side and back 8×, L leg kicks side and back 8×

Skate kick with pumping arms

R leg kicks forward and back 8×, L leg kicks forward and back 8×

High kick, travel backward and forward

Jumping jacks, travel sideways

Skate kick, travel backward and forward

(B set)

Cross-country ski

Cross-country ski, suspended

Tuck ski

Jacks tuck

Tuck ski and jacks tuck, alternate

Cross-country ski, suspended

Cross-country ski

(C set)

Knee-high jog, travel backward and forward

Squat with breaststroke and reverse breaststroke, alternate

Sprint

Knee-high jog, travel sideways

Squat with hand flutters

Sprint

(D set)

Jump rope, travel backward and forward (low-impact option: knee lift, big step, travel backward and forward)

Bunny hop, hands clasped behind back, travel backward and forward (low-impact option: walk with hands clasped behind back, travel backward and forward)

Log jump, forward and back (low-impact option: neutral position)

Log jump, side to side (low-impact option: neutral position)

Jacks tuck

Log jump one side, and jacks tuck, alternate

COOL-DOWN

(Noodle in hands)

Abdominal pike and spine extension

Side-to-side extension

Extension forward, R, back, L, and reverse

(Noodle behind shoulders)

Mermaid

Seated flutter kick

Hip curl with one foot on top of the other

Seated leg lift with one foot on top of the other

Teaser (Pilates)

Stretch: lower back, obliques, shoulders, hip flexors, gastrocnemius, neck

▶ **Shallow-Water Lesson Plan 10**

SHALLOW-WATER RUNNING

CLASS OBJECTIVE

Cardiorespiratory fitness

EQUIPMENT

None

TEACHING TIP

The arm moves sometimes assist and sometimes resist travel, decreasing and increasing the intensity. Running around the perimeter of the pool area sometimes creates a whirlpool effect in shallow water. If you have four lap lanes, try having participants run up lanes 1 and 3 and down lanes 2 and 4. They can also run back and forth, in a scatter pattern, or even in a figure eight.

WARM-UP

Instructor's choice

CONDITIONING PHASE

(A set)

Knee-high jog with breaststroke

Knee-high jog with reverse breaststroke

Knee-high jog with pumping arms

Knee-high jog, faster

(B set)

Knee-high jog with crawl stroke

Knee-high jog, push forward

Knee-high jog with pumping arms

Knee-high jog, faster

(C set)

Knee-high jog with jog press in front

Knee-high jog with jog press at sides

Knee-high jog with pumping arms

Knee-high jog, faster

Sprint

(D set)

Knee-high jog with lat pull-down

Knee-high jog with double-arm press-down

Knee-high jog with pumping arms

Knee-high jog, faster

Sprint

(E set)
Knee-high jog with arm swing
Knee-high jog with windshield wiper arms
Knee-high jog with pumping arms
Knee-high jog, faster

(F set)
Knee-high jog with arm curl
Knee-high jog with triceps extension
Knee-high jog with pumping arms
Knee-high jog, faster

(G set)
Knee-high jog with resistor arms
Knee-high jog with paddlewheel
Knee-high jog with pumping arms
Knee-high jog, faster
Sprint

(H set)
Knee-high jog, clap hands
Knee-high jog with shoulder blade squeeze
Knee-high jog with pumping arms
Knee-high jog, faster
Sprint

(I set)
Knee-high jog with forearm press
Knee-high jog, scull arms down
Knee-high jog with pumping arms
Knee-high jog, faster

(J set)
Knee-high jog with hands on hips
Knee-high jog with hands behind back
Knee-high jog with pumping arms
Knee-high jog, travel sideways

(K set)
Run tires, travel sideways
Kick side to side, travel sideways
Jumping jacks, travel sideways
Rocking horse to the side, travel sideways
Crab walk sideways
Step sideways, palms touch overhead
Squat, travel sideways

COOL-DOWN
Knee-high jog, pause on one foot with posture check
Walk forward with arms folded and legs straight
Ankle touch with double arms
Side crunch, standing
Hip hike
Stand on one foot and extend leg, hands up
Stretch: gastrocnemius, quadriceps, hip flexors, hamstrings, outer thigh, shoulders

▶ Shallow-Water Lesson Plan 11

TRAVEL

CLASS OBJECTIVE
Cardiorespiratory fitness

EQUIPMENT
Noodles

TEACHING TIP
Travel makes maximum use of the water's resistance.

WARM-UP
Instructor's choice

CONDITIONING PHASE
(A set)
Knee-high jog; travel backward, forward, and sideways
Knee-high jog, one knee only, travel sideways
Run tires; travel backward, forward, and sideways
Sprint

(B set)
Kick forward, push forward, travel backward and forward
Kick forward, neutral position, travel backward and forward
Jump flutter (low-impact option: seated flutter kick suspended)
High kick, travel backward and forward
Jump backward and leap forward (low-impact option: jump backward and sprint forward)
Skate kick with pumping arms, travel backward and forward

(C set)
Cross-country ski; travel backward, forward, and sideways

Cross-country ski, suspended

Jumping jacks, clap hands, travel backward and forward

Jumping jacks, travel sideways

Jacks cross

(D set)

Kick side to side; travel backward, forward, and sideways

Leap sideways (low-impact option: crab walk sideways)

Rocking horse to the side, travel sideways

Rocking horse with front kick

Rocking horse, travel backward and forward

Heel jog with crawl stroke, travel backward and forward

Two steps forward, side, back, side

COOL-DOWN

(Straddle noodle)

Bicycle with reverse breaststroke and no hands, travel backward and forward

Seated kick, travel backward and forward

Seated reverse breaststroke and breaststroke, travel backward and forward

Seated flutter kick with unison arm swing, travel backward and forward

(Noodle behind shoulders)

Bicycle, side-lying, travel

Tuck ski together, side-lying, travel

Cross-country ski, side-lying, travel

Hip curl, L position

Crunch, V position

Eight short crunches and two long crunches

(Hold noodle in hands)

Abdominal pike and spine extension

Stretch: quadriceps, gastrocnemius, hamstrings, outer thigh, inner thigh, obliques

▶ Shallow-Water Lesson Plan 12

TRAVEL WITH INTERVALS

CLASS OBJECTIVE

Cardiorespiratory fitness

EQUIPMENT

Noodles

TEACHING TIP

The resistance of traveling offers the potential for burning extra calories. Interval training improves cardiorespiratory fitness. A class that combines travel with intervals is good for participants who are trying to lose weight.

WARM-UP

Knee-high jog with jog press

Ankle touch

Hopscotch

Kick side to side

Kick forward, push forward

Rocking horse

CONDITIONING PHASE

(A set)

Knee-high jog, scull arms down, travel backward and forward

Knee-high jog with unison arm swing, travel backward and forward

Knee-high jog with breaststroke, travel backward and forward

Knee-high jog, palms touch in back, travel backward and forward

Interval high-intensity phase: cross-country ski, faster

Interval active recovery phase: cross-country ski

Interval high-intensity phase: ankle touch, faster

Interval active recovery phase: ankle touch

Interval high-intensity phase: mini ski, faster

Interval active recovery phase: cross-country ski

(B set)

Knee-high jog, pause on one foot with posture check

Sprint with hands fisted and cupped

Sprint with resistor arms; sprint, travel in a zigzag

Knee-high jog, travel in a scatter pattern

Interval high-intensity phase: cross-country ski, full ROM

Interval active recovery phase: cross-country ski

Interval high-intensity phase: jacks cross, full ROM

Interval active recovery phase: jumping jacks

Interval high-intensity phase: high kick

Interval active recovery phase: kick forward

(C set)

Cross-country ski, travel backward and forward

Jumping jacks, clap hands, travel backward and forward

High kick, travel backward; skate kick, travel forward

Hopscotch, travel backward and forward

Interval high-intensity phase: cross-country ski, suspended

Interval active recovery phase: cross-country ski, neutral position

Interval high-intensity phase: jumping jacks, suspended

Interval active recovery phase: jumping jacks, neutral position

Interval high-intensity phase: bicycle, suspended

Interval active recovery phase: knee-high jog, neutral position

(D set)

Cross-country ski, travel sideways

Jumping jacks, travel sideways

Rocking horse to the side, travel sideways

Crab walk sideways

Interval high-intensity phase: cross-country ski with power

Interval active recovery phase: cross-country ski

Interval high-intensity phase: kick side to side, arms and legs opposite, with power

Interval active recovery phase: kick side to side

Interval high-intensity phase: steep climb

Interval active recovery phase: knee-high jog

COOL-DOWN

(Straddle noodle)

Seated kick, travel backward and forward

Seated jacks, travel backward and forward

Seated reverse breaststroke and breaststroke, travel backward and forward

(Noodle behind shoulders)

Hip curl from a kneeling position

Side crunch from a kneeling position

Side-to-side extension

Side-to-side extension, doubles

V-sit

Hold V and scull to travel forward

Stretch: shoulders, upper back, pectorals, quadriceps, hamstrings, inner thigh, outer thigh

▶ Shallow-Water Lesson Plan 13

TRAVEL UPRIGHT, NEUTRAL POSITION AND SUSPENDED

CLASS OBJECTIVE

Cardiorespiratory fitness

EQUIPMENT

Noodles

TEACHING TIP

Travel in the neutral position increases resistance because more of the body is underwater. Travel suspended makes use of two ways to increase intensity.

WARM-UP

Knee-high jog with jog press

Straddle jog with shoulder blade squeeze

Knee-high jog, palms touch in back

Walk forward

Walk backward

Crossover step

Crab walk sideways

CONDITIONING PHASE

(A set) (intensity level 1)

Knee-high jog, hands fisted, travel forward (1 min.)

Knee-high jog, scull in front, travel backward (1 min.)

Kick forward with unison arm swing, travel forward (1 min.)

Jumping jacks, travel backward (1 min.)

Knee-high jog, hands cupped, travel forward (1 min.)

Jump backward (1 min.)

Jumping jacks, neutral position, travel forward (1 min.)

Kick forward, neutral position, travel backward (1 min.)

(B set) (intensity level 2)

Knee-high jog with breaststroke, travel forward (1 min.)

Straddle jog, clap hands, travel backward (1 min.)

Cross-country ski, suspended, travel forward (1 min.)

Jump backward (1 min.)

Bicycle, suspended, travel forward (1 min.)

Knee-high jog with reverse breaststroke, travel backward (1 min.)

Bicycle, suspended, travel forward (1 min.)

Jumping jacks, neutral position, travel backward (1 min.)

Cross-country ski, travel forward (1 min.)

Knee-high jog, push forward, travel backward (1 min.)

Cross-country ski, travel forward (1 min.)

High kick, neutral position, travel backward (1 min.)

Jumping jacks, clap hands, travel forward (1 min.)

High kick, travel backward (1 min.)

Frog jump, travel forward (low-impact option: neutral position) (1 min.)

Jumping jacks, neutral position, travel backward (1 min.)

(C set) (intensity level 1)

Knee-high jog, hands fisted, travel forward (1 min.)

Knee-high jog, scull in front, travel backward (1 min.)

Kick forward with unison arm swing, travel forward (1 min.)

Jumping jacks, travel backward (1 min.)

Knee-high jog, hands cupped, travel forward (1 min.)

Jump backward (1 min.)

Jumping jacks, neutral position, travel forward (1 min.)

Kick forward, neutral position, travel backward (1 min.)

COOL-DOWN

(Noodle behind shoulders)

Cross-country ski, side-lying

Bicycle, side-lying, in a circle

Side-to-side extension

Seated leg lift, hold for 15 seconds

Stand on noodle and balance with one leg lifted forward

Stand on noodle and balance with one leg extended backward

Stretch: gastrocnemius, quadriceps, hamstrings, outer thigh, hip flexors, shoulders

▶ Shallow-Water Lesson Plan 14

TRAVEL UPRIGHT AND SEATED WITH NOODLES

CLASS OBJECTIVE

Muscular strength and endurance

EQUIPMENT

Noodles

TEACHING TIP

Noodles can be used as resistance equipment for the upper body and as flotation support for lower-body strength training.

WARM-UP

Instructor's choice

CONDITIONING PHASE

(A set)

Kick forward with standing row with noodle, travel backward and forward

Kick forward, push noodle down on one side, travel sideways

Seated kick, feet pointed, sit on noodle like a swing, travel backward

Heel jog, swing noodle side to side, travel backward and forward

Heel jog, push noodle down in front, travel sideways

Seated kick, feet flexed, sit on noodle like a swing, travel forward

Knee-high jog, touch ends of noodle in back

Power run, noodle under chest

(B set)

Rocking horse, push noodle down in front, travel backward and forward

Rocking horse, scoop noodle out to the side, travel sideways

Seated flutter kick, sit on noodle like a swing

Cross-country ski, push forward, hold ends of noodle, travel backward and forward

Cross-country ski, noodle in one hand, travel sideways

High kick, straddle noodle, travel backward and forward

Knee-high jog, push noodle forward, down, and up

Power run, noodle under chest

(C set)

Jumping jacks, touch ends of noodle in front, travel backward and forward

Jumping jacks, noodle in one hand, travel sideways

Seated jacks, straddle noodle, travel backward and forward

Straddle jog with double-arm press-down, hold ends of noodle together, travel backward and forward

Straddle jog, hold noodle overhead, travel sideways

Seated leg press, straddle noodle, travel backward and forward

Knee-high jog with forearm press, noodle around waist

Power run, noodle under chest

COOL-DOWN

Knee-high jog, noodle in a paddlewheel, travel backward and forward

Bicycle, side-lying, noodle behind shoulders, travel

Bicycle, straddle noodle, travel backward and forward

(Stand on noodle)

Use as a stair climber

Balance with one leg extended backward

Hop; travel backward, forward, and sideways

Hop with one leg lifted forward

Hop with one leg extended backward

Stretch: upper back, pectorals, latissimus dorsi, triceps, shoulders, quadriceps, hamstrings

▶ Shallow-Water Lesson Plan 15

ALL-NOODLE WORKOUT

CLASS OBJECTIVE

Muscular strength and endurance

EQUIPMENT

Noodles

TEACHING TIP

Spice up your class occasionally with an all-noodle workout. The partner moves add fun.

WARM-UP

(Hold noodle in hands)

Knee-high jog

Straddle jog

Side quad kick

Jumping jacks

Kick forward

Heel jog

CONDITIONING PHASE

(A set)

Knee-high jog, push noodle forward

Knee-high jog with standing row

Rocking horse, push noodle down

Jumping jacks, noodle in one hand, travel sideways

Jumping jacks, touch ends of noodle in front

Push-ups

Cross-country ski, noodle in R hand, travel sideways

Power run, noodle under chest

Cross-country ski, noodle in L hand, travel sideways

Power run, noodle under chest

Cross-country ski with one foot on noodle

Jumping jacks with one foot on noodle

Jumping jacks, touch ends of noodle in front

Push-ups

Knee-high jog with double-arm press-down, hold ends of noodle together, travel backward

Knee-high jog with double-arm lift, hold ends of noodle together, travel forward

Jumping jacks with forearm press, noodle around waist

(B set) (Straddle noodle)

High kick

Ankle touch

Bicycle, reverse, travel backward; and bicycle, tandem, travel forward

Seated reverse breaststroke and breaststroke, travel backward and forward

(C set) (Noodle behind shoulders)

Cross-country ski, side-lying, travel

Tuck ski together, side-lying, travel

Knee-high jog, side-lying, travel

Bicycle, side-lying, travel

(D set)

Partner cross-country ski (partners hold opposite ends of two noodles)

Partner jumping jacks

Partner ski–jacks combo (Cue: *ski, ski, jack, together*)

Tug of war (partners back to back, hold ends of both noodles under arms and run in opposite directions)

Partner bicycle in a circle (partners back to back, noodles behind shoulders and linked)

Bicycle races (partner 1 runs with noodle in front and under arms; partner 2 straddles a noodle and bicycles holding ends of partner 1's noodle)

Rickshaw (partner 1 runs holding ends of noodles under arms; partner 2 floats in a seated position holding opposite ends)

Canoe races (straddle noodle and paddle with arms)

COOL-DOWN

(Noodle under chest)

Rock climb

(Noodle in hands)

Abdominal pike and spine extension

Side-to-side extension

(Stand on noodle)

Standing leg press with one foot on noodle

Use as a stair climber

Surf

Balance with one leg lifted forward

Balance with one leg extended backward

Stretch: upper back, pectorals, obliques, triceps, gastrocnemius, hip flexors, outer thigh

VARIATIONS ON A THEME

Variations on a theme is a type of linear choreography. Instead of using many different exercises, though, you limit yourself to two or three basic exercises and work these through multiple variations. The choreography can be represented by the letters a1, a2, a3, b1, b2, b3. For example, in Shallow-Water Lesson Plan 16, "a" is knee-high jog and "b" is run tires, and the numbers 1, 2, 3 are the variations:

a. Knee-high jog, with 1. Upper-body twist

a. Knee-high jog, with 2. Elbows together

a. Knee-high jog, with 3. Speed and a longer stride (Sprint)

b. Run tires, with 1. Jog press in front

b. Run tires, with 2. Clap hands

b. Run tires, with 3. Speed (faster)

If you would like to try writing your own variations on a theme, begin by selecting your basic exercises. You want to use exercises that work different muscle groups to avoid the fatigue that would come from using a single muscle group for an entire class. An example is to use cross-country ski, which works the legs front to back, and jumping jacks, which work the legs to the sides. What arm moves can you add to the leg moves? Some arm moves slice, reducing resistance, and some have the palms face the direction of motion, increasing resistance. Try changing the working positions from upright to neutral to suspended. Have participants travel forward, backward, or sideways in the various working positions. Add intensity by increasing speed, range of motion, or power, or decrease intensity by having participants slow down, make the move smaller, or back off from pushing hard against the water. Can you change the move to cross the midline of the body, or combine it with another move? Thinking about all the ways to change an exercise will help you come up with your own variations on a theme.

▶ Shallow-Water Lesson Plan 16

KNEE AND HEEL

CLASS OBJECTIVE

Cardiorespiratory fitness

EQUIPMENT

Noodles

TEACHING TIP

Be sure to cue good posture in the neutral position. Some participants tend to round their shoulders when they work low in the water.

WARM-UP

Knee-high jog with jog press

Knee-high jog with shoulder blade squeeze

Run tires with scull

Run tires, reach to the sides

Heel jog, palms touch in back

Heel jog with triceps extension

Rocking horse

CONDITIONING PHASE

(A set)

Knee-high jog with upper-body twist

Knee-high jog, elbows together

Knee-high jog, faster

Run tires with jog press in front

Run tires, clap hands

Run tires, faster

Heel jog with jog press

Heel jog with lat pull-down

Heel jog, faster

Rocking horse with arm curl

Rocking horse with shoulder blade squeeze

Rocking horse, faster

(B set)

Knee-high jog

Jump rope (low-impact option: log jump, forward and back, neutral position)

Knee-high jog, neutral position

Hip curl, suspended

Run tires

Frog jump (low-impact option: neutral position)

Run tires, neutral position

Diamond position, open and close knees, suspended

Heel jog

Bunny hop (low-impact option: heel jog, doubles)

Skip rope

Skateboard jump

Rocking horse with front kick

(C set)

Knee-high jog

Knee lift and lunge

Knee-high jog, one knee only, travel sideways

Ankle touch

Run tires

In in, out out

Heel jog

Heel jog, one heel only, travel sideways

Heel jog, feet wide apart

Hopscotch

Ankle touch and hopscotch, alternate

Ankle touch and hopscotch, one side only

(D set)

Knee-high jog; travel backward, forward, and sideways

Sprint

Run tires; travel backward, forward, and sideways

Heel jog; travel backward, forward, and sideways

Rocking horse; travel backward, forward, and sideways

Ankle touch, travel backward; hopscotch, travel forward

Walk forward three steps and stand on one foot with posture check

COOL-DOWN

(Noodle behind shoulders)

Bicycle, side-lying, travel

Bicycle, side-lying, in a circle

Bicycle

Bicycle, one leg only

Bicycle, reverse

(Without noodles)

Abdominal pike and spine extension at the wall

Stretch: hip flexors, quadriceps, gastrocnemius, hamstrings, lower back, shoulders

▶ Shallow-Water Lesson Plan 17

CROSS-COUNTRY SKI AND JUMPING JACKS

CLASS OBJECTIVE
Cardiorespiratory fitness

EQUIPMENT
Noodles

TEACHING TIP
When focusing on variations of two exercises, be sure that participants stretch the muscle groups used in those two exercises at the end of the cooldown.

WARM-UP
Instructor's choice

CONDITIONING PHASE

(A set)
Cross-country ski
Cross-country ski, clap hands
Cross-country ski with unison arm swing
Cross-country ski with forearm press, side to side
Cross-country ski, faster
Jumping jacks
Jumping jacks, arms cross in front
Jumping jacks, arms cross in back
Jumping jacks, arms cross in front and back, alternate
Jumping jacks, faster

(B set)
Cross-country ski
Tuck ski
Cross-country ski, suspended
Cross-country ski
Jumping jacks
Air Jordan jacks (low-impact option: jumping jacks with power)
Jumping jacks, land with feet in only (low-impact option: neutral position)

Jumping jacks, land with feet out only (low-impact option: neutral position)
Jumping jacks, squat
Jacks tuck
Jumping jacks, suspended; travel backward, forward, and sideways

(C set)
Mini ski
Cross-country ski, full ROM
Mini jacks
Jacks cross, full ROM
Mini cross
Triple crossover

(D set)
Cross-country ski, corner to corner
Tuck ski
Tuck ski, corner to corner
Cross-country ski and jumping jacks, alternate
Ski R, jack, ski L, jack
Ski 3×, jack 1×
Jacks tuck
Tuck ski and jacks tuck, alternate

(E set)
Cross-country ski; travel backward, forward, and sideways
Cross-country ski with quarter turn
Cross-country ski 3 1/2×, half turn
Jumping jacks; travel backward, forward, and sideways
Jumping jacks with quarter turn
Jacks cross 3 1/2×, half turn

COOL-DOWN
(Noodle behind shoulders)
Seated Cossack kick
Seated jacks
Cross-country ski, side-lying
Side kick (Pilates)
Single-leg stretch (Pilates)
Double-leg stretch (Pilates)
Stretch: hamstrings, outer thigh, inner thigh, hip flexors, gastrocnemius, latissimus dorsi

Shallow-Water Lesson Plan 18

KICKS

CLASS OBJECTIVE
Cardiorespiratory fitness

EQUIPMENT
None

TEACHING TIP
Some participants tend to power pop the knees when kicking, which is hard on the knee joint. Cue soft knees.

WARM-UP
Kick forward with scull
Kick forward with arm swing
Kick side to side with arms extended to sides
Kick side to side with windshield wiper arms
Skate kick, scull arms down
Skate kick with pumping arms

CONDITIONING PHASE
(A set)
Kick forward, clap hands
Kick forward, faster
Kick side to side, arms cross in front
Kick side to side, faster
Skate kick, push forward
Skate kick, faster

(B set)
Kick forward
Kick forward, neutral position
Kick forward, suspended
Kick to the corners, neutral position
Kick to the corners, suspended
Cossack kick, neutral position
Jump backward
Leap forward (low-impact option: sprint forward)
High kick
Skate kick, higher
Kick side to side, arms sweep side to side
Skate kick with power

(C set)
Kick forward, travel backward and forward
High kick, travel backward and forward

Kick side to side; travel backward, forward, and sideways
Skate kick, travel backward and forward
Skip rope, travel backward and forward

(D set)
Chorus line kick
Quad kick
Front kick (karate)
Side kick (karate)
Side kick on one side, leg stays up
Kick forward
Kick to the corners
Kick forward and to the corners, alternate
Kick and lunge
In-line skate
Skip rope
One leg kicks forward and back
One leg—knee lift, kick forward, side knee lift, kick side, heel lift, kick back
One leg kicks forward, side, back, side

COOL-DOWN
Walk backward and lunge forward low in the water
Walk forward, hands up
Pelvic tilt, standing
Standing crunch
Heels out, then toes in
Heels wide on floor in front, then toes on floor in center, then toes wide on floor in back
Stretch: hip flexors, quadriceps, outer thigh, inner thigh, hamstrings, lower back

▶ **Shallow-Water Lesson Plan 19**

JOG AND WALK

CLASS OBJECTIVE
Cardiorespiratory fitness

EQUIPMENT
Noodles

TEACHING TIP
Try several different cues for good posture to get the idea across (e.g., *Ears over shoulders, shoulders over hips, feet under you; Chest up, shoulders back;*

Tuck the chin in; Walk as if you had a book on your head). For the arm medley, choose any upper-body moves you like.

WARM-UP

Knee-high jog

Straddle jog

Step sideways

Walk backward and forward

Walk 4×, jog 8×

CONDITIONING PHASE

(A set)

Knee-high jog

Knee-high jog, faster

Sprint

Straddle jog

Straddle jog, faster

(B set)

Knee-high jog with arm medley

(C set)

Knee-high jog

Squat and jump (low-impact option: jacks tuck, neutral position)

Knee-high jog, neutral position, travel backward and forward

Hip curl, suspended

Knee-high jog

Straddle jog

Frog jump, neutral position

Frog jump, neutral position, travel backward and forward

Frog jump, suspended

(D set)

Knee-high jog, one knee only, travel sideways

Knee-high jog; travel backward, forward, and sideways

Knee-high jog, faster

Sprint

Straddle jog; travel backward, forward, and sideways

(E set)

Knee-high jog

Knee lift and lunge

Knee-high jog with upper-body twist

Straddle jog with elbows to knees

In in, out out

Ankle touch, feet close together

Ankle touch, feet wide apart

Ankle touch, travel backward and forward

Hopscotch, feet close together

Hopscotch, feet wide apart

Hopscotch, travel backward and forward

(F set)

Walk on toes and walk on heels

Walk forward with arms folded and legs straight

Knee lift, big step; travel backward, forward, and sideways

Crossover step

Lunge forward, low in the water

Squat, travel sideways

Two steps forward, side, back, side

COOL-DOWN

(Noodle behind shoulders)

Crunch, V position

Seated flutter kick

Seated high kick

Seated jacks, toes in

Seated jacks, toes out

Flutter kick, side-lying

Stretch: gastrocnemius, hip flexors, quadriceps, hamstrings, outer thigh, upper back, neck

▶ Shallow-Water Lesson Plan 20

CROSS-COUNTRY SKI, JUMPING JACKS, AND JUMP

CLASS OBJECTIVE

Cardiorespiratory fitness

EQUIPMENT

Noodles

TEACHING TIP

You want your participants to land softly when they jump, so be sure to cue landing toe-ball-heel. Offer low-impact options for participants who should avoid jumping. For the arm medley, choose any upper-body moves you like.

WARM-UP

Knee-high jog

Knee-high jog, travel with arm medley

Knee-high jog, travel backward and forward in a zigzag

CONDITIONING PHASE

(A set)

Cross-country ski, hands slicing

Cross-country ski, palms face direction of motion

Cross-country ski, faster

Jumping jacks, arms cross in front and in back

Jumping jacks, palms touch in front and in back

Jumping jacks, faster

Bunny hop (low-impact option: log jump, forward and back, neutral position)

Jump flutter (low-impact option: log jump, side to side, neutral position)

(B set)

Cross-country ski, neutral position, travel backward and forward

Cross-country ski, suspended

Jumping jacks, neutral position, travel backward and forward

Jumping jacks, suspended

Squat and jump (low-impact option: jacks tuck, neutral position)

Hip curl, suspended

Basketball jump (low-impact option: frog jump, neutral position)

(C set)

Cross-country ski with power

Jumping jacks with power

Bicycle, climb a hill, suspended

(D set)

Crossover kick

Cross-country ski, corner to corner

Skate kick

Jacks cross

Mini cross

Triple crossover

Ankle touch

Ankle touch, one ankle only

Hopscotch

Hopscotch, one heel only

Log jump, forward and back (low-impact option: neutral position)

Log jump, side to side (low-impact option: neutral position)

Jump in a circle and reverse (low-impact option: neutral position)

Knee-high jog

Skateboard

Knee-high jog with quick change of direction

(E set)

Cross-country ski, travel backward and forward

Jumping jacks, travel sideways

Jump backward and leap forward (low-impact option: jump backward and sprint forward)

Knee-high jog, follow the leader

Knee-high jog, travel in a scatter pattern

Lunge forward, low in the water

COOL-DOWN

(Noodle in hands)

Diamond fall forward, tuck and stand

Side fall, tuck and stand

Abdominal pike and spine extension with legs in a diamond position

(Noodle behind shoulders)

Side-to-side extension with legs in a diamond position

Crunch, with legs in a diamond position

Hip curl, with legs in a diamond position

Stretch: hamstrings, inner thigh, outer thigh, quadriceps, hip flexors, gastrocnemius

ADD-ON CHOREOGRAPHY

Add-on choreography is another type of choreography that is easy to write. It is called "add-on" because after you teach a set of exercises, you add on a second set. Repeat those two sets and then add on a third set. Continue the pattern, adding a new set each time around. Add-on choreography can be represented by the letters AB, ABC, ABCD, and so on. You will need five to seven sets of exercises with four to six exercises in each set for a typical class. Select exercises that work well together. The exercises may work well together because they are similar types (e.g., kicks); they all work the body in the same direction (e.g., front to back); or they set up a simple travel pattern (e.g., travel backward with one exercise and forward with another). If you decide to include travel, allow enough time for your participants to move from one end of the area to the other. Use your creativity in putting sets together and you will soon have lots of ideas for add-on choreography.

▶ Shallow-Water Lesson Plan 21

ADD-ON CHOREOGRAPHY 1

CLASS OBJECTIVE
Cardiorespiratory fitness

EQUIPMENT
None

TEACHING TIP
Have participants perform each exercise 16 times the first time you teach a set; then you can pick up the pace if you like by having them perform the exercises 8 times, or even 4 times, the next time around. When you move on to the next exercise quickly, it is more challenging to keep up.

WARM-UP
Instructor's choice

CONDITIONING PHASE
(A set)
Kick forward
Kick to the corners
Kick side to side
Cross-country ski

(B set)
Kick forward
In-line skate
Quad kick
One leg kicks forward and back

(Repeat A and B and add C set)
Ankle touch
Hopscotch
Side quad kick
Ankle touch and hopscotch, alternate

(Repeat A–C and add D set)
Crossover knees
Crossover kick
High kick

(Repeat A–D and add E set)
Skateboard
Cross-country ski
Cross-country ski 3 1/2×, half turn
Mini ski

(Repeat A–E and add F set)
Hitchhike
Jacks cross
Jacks cross 3 1/2×, half turn
Mini jacks

(Repeat A–F and add G set)
Knee-high jog
Heel jog
Rocking horse
Skateboard jump

COOL-DOWN
Heels out, then toes in
Heels out, then chair position suspended, then L position, then chair position suspended
Heels wide on floor in front, then toes on floor in center, then toes wide on floor in back
Abdominal pike and spine extension with no equipment
Upper-body twist
Lower-body twist
Hula hoop
Stretch: quadriceps, gastrocnemius, hamstrings, outer thigh, obliques, shoulders

▶ Shallow-Water Lesson Plan 22

ADD-ON CHOREOGRAPHY 2

CLASS OBJECTIVES
Cardiorespiratory fitness and muscular strength and endurance

EQUIPMENT
Noodles

TEACHING TIP

Try strength training by having participants use noodles for resistance during the cool-down. Then have them stand on the noodles for balance training.

WARM-UP

Instructor's choice

CONDITIONING PHASE

(A set)
Jumping jacks 4× and turn 4×
Sprint
Cross-country ski, travel backward
Kick forward, travel forward

(B set)
Jump backward
Rocking horse R, travel sideways
Jacks tuck, travel backward
Rocking horse L, travel sideways

(Repeat A and B and add C set)
Heel jog, travel backward
Skate kick, travel forward
Repeat

(Repeat A–C and add D set)
Rocking horse, R foot forward
Skateboard jump, R foot forward
Cross-country ski, suspended
Repeat set with L foot forward

(Repeat A–D and add E set)
Jumping jacks, clap hands, travel backward
Sprint, travel in a zigzag
Cross-country ski, travel backward
Sprint with resistor arms

COOL-DOWN

(Noodle in hands)
Standing row, squat position
Push noodle forward, squat position
Push noodle down in front, squat position
Push noodle down on one side, squat position
Touch ends of noodle in front with jumping jacks
Double-arm press-down, hold ends of noodle together, squat position

Touch ends of noodle in back with jumping jacks
Forearm press, noodle around waist, with jumping jacks
(Stand on noodle)
Hop; travel backward, forward, and sideways
Balance with one leg extended backward
Hop with one leg lifted forward
Hop with one leg extended backward
Stretch: lower back, hamstrings, outer thigh, upper back, pectorals, triceps, shoulders

▶ **Shallow-Water Lesson Plan 23**

ADD-ON CHOREOGRAPHY 3

CLASS OBJECTIVE

Cardiorespiratory fitness

EQUIPMENT

Noodles

TEACHING TIP

You can alternate two exercises to increase intensity. Have participants do four repetitions of each pair of exercises in sets C and D, alternating back and forth three times.

WARM-UP

Instructor's choice

CONDITIONING PHASE

(A set)
Jumping jacks, clap hands, travel backward
Rocking horse R, travel forward
Skateboard R
Jump backward
Rocking horse L, travel forward
Skateboard L

(B set)
Leap sideways (low-impact option: squat, travel sideways)
Sprint
Rocking horse, circle R
Leap sideways (low-impact option: squat, travel sideways)
Sprint
Rocking horse, circle L

(Repeat A and B and add C set)

Knee-high jog and cross-country ski, corner to corner; alternate 3×

Knee-high jog, faster and tuck ski; alternate 3×

Knee-high jog and high kick, alternate 3×

Knee-high jog, faster and frog jump; alternate 3×

(Repeat A–C and add D set)

Hopscotch and skate kick, alternate 3×

Ankle touch and jacks cross, alternate 3×

Steep climb and bicycle, suspended; alternate 3×

(Repeat A–D and add E set)

Kick and lunge R, cross-country ski, kick and lunge L

Side kick (karate) R, kick side to side, side kick (karate) L

Cross-country ski and jumping jacks, alternate

Kick forward; seated kick, travel backward; kick forward, suspended, travel forward

COOL-DOWN

(Noodle behind shoulders)

Crunch, V position

V-sit

Hold V and scull to travel forward

Cross-country ski, side-lying

Side kick (Pilates)

Stretch: outer thigh, inner thigh, hamstrings, quadriceps, latissimus dorsi, obliques

BLOCK CHOREOGRAPHY

Block choreography is more complex than linear or add-on choreography, but once you get the pattern down, you will be able to come up with many variations. One way to write block choreography is to begin by writing a 10-minute sample class. What will you include? You have many options to choose from such as intervals, travel, upper-body moves, working in a neutral position, one-sided moves, doubles, and combining two moves. Your 10-minute sample class is your first set. What can you change for the second set? If you used intervals, can you think of a different way to increase intensity? If you used travel, can you have participants travel in a different direction? If you used upper-body moves, can you think of exercises for a different muscle group? The changes

you make to your 10-minute sample class are your second set. Repeat the process two more times, and you have written a 40-minute conditioning set. Block choreography can be represented by the letters a1, b1, c1, d1; a2, b2, c2, d2; a3, b3, c3, d3, and so on. Look, for example, at the two sample sets below. The exercises in the first set are repeated with variations in the second set.

(A set)

(a1) Rocking horse

(b1) Heel jog with shoulder blade squeeze

(c1) Skip rope

(d1) Cross-country ski

(e1) Jumping jacks

(B set)

(a2) Rocking horse with front kick (add front kick)

(b2) Heel jog, clap hands (different arm move)

(c2) Skip rope, travel backward and forward (add travel)

(d2) Cross-country ski, corner to corner (cross midline of body)

(e2) Jacks cross (increase ROM)

You don't have to change everything in your block choreography sets. You may wish to begin each set with the same three exercises, repeat a move from the first set in the third set, or have more sets of fewer exercises. Once you get started, the variations are endless.

▶ Shallow-Water Lesson Plan 24

UPRIGHT AND SEATED MOVES

CLASS OBJECTIVE

Cardiorespiratory fitness

EQUIPMENT

Noodles

TEACHING TIP

The sets begin with cross-country ski and a variation of cross-country ski. Then each set features a different exercise adding an upper-body move, travel, and intervals. The cool-down repeats all the moves in a seated position using noodles for flotation.

WARM-UP

Instructor's choice

CONDITIONING PHASE

(A set)

Cross-country ski

Cross-country ski, suspended

Kick forward with shoulder blade squeeze

Kick forward, travel backward and forward

Interval high-intensity phase: high kick

Interval active recovery phase: kick forward

(B set)

Cross-country ski

Cross-country ski, corner to corner

Heel jog with standing row

Heel jog, travel backward and forward

Interval high-intensity phase: bunny hop (low-impact option: hitchhike, faster)

Interval active recovery phase: heel jog

(C set)

Cross-country ski

Mini ski

Skate kick with lat pull-down

Skate kick, travel backward and forward

Interval high-intensity phase: skate kick with power

Interval active recovery phase: skate kick

(D set)

Cross-country ski

Cross-country ski, neutral position, full ROM

Jumping jacks with elbows bent

Jumping jacks, travel backward and forward

Interval high-intensity phase: jumping jacks, faster

Interval active recovery phase: jumping jacks

(E set)

Cross-country ski

Tuck ski

Run tires with arm curl, palms face direction of motion

Run tires, travel backward and forward

Interval high-intensity phase: squat and jump (low-impact option: frog jump, suspended)

Interval active recovery phase: run tires

(F set)

Cross-country ski

Tuck ski, corner to corner

Knee-high jog with unison jog press

Knee-high jog, travel backward and forward

Interval high-intensity phase: steep climb

Interval active recovery phase: knee-high jog

COOL-DOWN

(Noodle behind shoulders)

Seated kick, feet pointed

Seated kick, feet flexed

Seated high kick

Seated jacks

Seated leg press

Bicycle

Bicycle, side-lying, travel

Tuck ski together, side-lying, travel

Stretch: pectorals, upper back, lower back, hamstrings, outer thigh, gastrocnemius

▶ Shallow-Water Lesson Plan 25

UPPER BODY AND SPRINTS

CLASS OBJECTIVES

Cardiorespiratory fitness and muscular strength and endurance

EQUIPMENT

Noodles

TEACHING TIP

Each set includes upper-body strength training exercises focusing on different muscle groups performed while the legs move to stay warm. Finish off the set with sprints the length of the pool to bring heart rates into the upper level of the target heart rates; then use an exercise in the neutral position for the active recovery. The last exercise before stretching is rolling like a ball. If you have participants who feel uncomfortable reclining with a noodle under the knees, you may want to skip this exercise.

WARM-UP

Instructor's choice

CONDITIONING PHASE

(A set)

One leg kicks forward and back

High kick

Ankle touch

Knee-high jog with crossovers

Knee-high jog with chest fly

Knee-high jog with shoulder blade squeeze

Knee-high jog with standing row

Knee-high jog, clap hands, travel backward and forward

Sprint

Tuck ski

(B set)

One leg kicks forward and back

Skate kick

Hopscotch

Jumping jacks, palms touch in front

Jumping jacks, palms touch in back

Jumping jacks, palms touch in front and back

Jumping jacks with lat pull-down with elbows bent

Jumping jacks with double-arm press-down, travel backward and forward

Sprint 2 laps

Jacks tuck

(C set)

One leg kicks forward and back

High kick

Ankle touch

Knee-high jog, open and close doors

Knee-high jog with arm curl

Knee-high jog with triceps extension

Knee-high jog with unison jog press, travel backward and forward

Sprint 3 laps

Frog jump, neutral position

(D set)

One leg kicks forward and back

Skate kick

Hopscotch

Knee-high jog with scull

Knee-high jog with hand flutters

Knee-high jog with paddlewheel and reverse

Knee-high jog with forearm press, travel backward and forward

Sprint, travel in a scatter pattern

Knee-high jog, travel in a scatter pattern

Jump in a circle

COOL-DOWN

(Noodle behind shoulders)

Crunch with legs in a diamond position

Hip curl with legs in a diamond position

Seated leg lift, hold for 15 seconds

Side-to-side extension with legs in a diamond position

(Noodle under knees)

Rolling like a ball (Pilates)

Stretch: upper back, pectorals, latissimus dorsi, triceps, shoulders, gastrocnemius

▶ Shallow-Water Lesson Plan 26

INTERVALS WITH KNEE-HIGH JOG

CLASS OBJECTIVE

Cardiorespiratory fitness

EQUIPMENT

Noodles

TEACHING TIP

There are many ways to do intervals. One way is to use a single exercise such as knee-high jog and use different ways of increasing intensity in each set of block choreography.

WARM-UP

Instructor's choice

CONDITIONING PHASE

(A set)

Knee-high jog with shoulder blade squeeze

Knee-high jog with reverse breaststroke and breaststroke, travel backward and forward

Cross-country ski, travel backward and forward

Jumping jacks, clap hands, travel backward and forward

Mini jacks

Jacks tuck
Cossack kick, neutral position
Interval high-intensity phase: knee-high jog, faster
Interval active recovery phase: knee-high jog

(B set)
Knee-high jog with arm lift to sides
Knee-high jog with double-arm press-down, travel backward and forward
Cross-country ski, travel sideways
Jumping jacks, travel sideways
Jacks cross
Jacks tuck
Frog jump (low-impact option: neutral position)
Interval high-intensity phase: leap forward (low-impact option: sprint)
Interval active recovery phase: knee-high jog

(C set)
Knee-high jog with arm curl, palms face direction of motion
Knee-high jog, push forward, travel backward and forward
Cross-country ski, travel backward and forward
Jumping jacks, clap hands, travel backward and forward
Mini cross
Jacks tuck
Log jump, side to side (low-impact option: neutral position)
Interval high-intensity phase: knee-high jog, suspended
Interval active recovery phase: knee-high jog, neutral position

(D set)
Knee-high jog with unison jog press
Knee-high jog with forearm press, travel backward and forward
Cross-country ski, travel sideways
Jumping jacks, travel sideways
Jumping jacks, squat
Jacks tuck
Heels out, then toes in

Interval high-intensity phase: steep climb
Interval active recovery phase: knee-high jog

COOL-DOWN
(Noodle in hands)
Abdominal pike and spine extension
Diamond fall forward, tuck and stand
Side fall, tuck and stand
(Stand on noodle)
Use as a stair climber
Surf
Surf with reverse breaststroke and breaststroke, travel backward and forward
Stretch: gastrocnemius, hip flexors, quadriceps, hamstrings, shoulders, neck

▶ **Shallow-Water Lesson Plan 27**

INTERVALS WITH KICK FORWARD

CLASS OBJECTIVE
Cardiorespiratory fitness

EQUIPMENT
Noodles

TEACHING TIP
Participants sweat during water aerobics but may not realize it because of the cooling effect of the water. Encourage them to drink water. For the arm medley, choose any upper-body moves you like.

WARM-UP
Instructor's choice

CONDITIONING PHASE
(A set)
Kick forward with shoulder blade squeeze
Knee-high jog, palms touch in back
Run tires, reach to the sides
Rocking horse to the side
Cross-country ski, travel backward and forward
Cross-country ski
Jumping jacks
Interval high-intensity phase: kick forward, faster
Interval active recovery phase: kick forward
Knee-high jog

(B set)

Kick forward with reverse breaststroke and breaststroke, travel backward and forward

Knee-high jog, one knee only, travel sideways

Run tires, travel sideways

Rocking horse to the side, travel sideways

Jumping jacks, clap hands, travel backward and forward

Jacks cross

Cross-country ski, corner to corner

Interval high-intensity phase: high kick

Interval active recovery phase: kick forward

Knee-high jog

(C set)

Kick forward with reverse breaststroke, travel backward and forward

Jump rope, arms circle forward (low impact option: skip rope, arms circle forward)

Run tires, travel backward and forward

Rocking horse with front kick

Cross-country ski, travel sideways

Tuck ski

Jumping jacks, squat

Interval high-intensity phase: kick forward, suspended

Interval active recovery phase: kick forward, neutral position

Knee-high jog

(D set)

Knee-high jog with arm medley

(E set)

Kick forward with breaststroke, travel backward and forward

Jump rope, arms circle backward (low impact option: skip rope, arms circle backward)

Frog jump (low-impact option: neutral position)

Rocking horse with shoulder blade squeeze

Jumping jacks, travel sideways

Mini cross

Tuck ski, corner to corner

Jump backward and kick forward, travel forward

Knee-high jog

COOL-DOWN

(Noodle in hands)

Abdominal pike and spine extension

Abdominal pike and spine extension, legs wide in front and together in back

Abdominal pike and spine extension, legs together in front and wide in back

Abdominal pike and spine extension, legs wide in front and wide in back with tuck in center

Stretch: hip flexors, quadriceps, hamstrings, upper back, pectorals, shoulders

▶ Shallow-Water Lesson Plan 28

INTERVALS WITH CROSS-COUNTRY SKI

CLASS OBJECTIVE

Cardiorespiratory fitness

EQUIPMENT

Noodles

TEACHING TIP

Cross-country ski works well with all of the ways to increase intensity, which makes it a good exercise to use in interval training. For the arm medley, choose any upper-body moves you like.

WARM-UP

Instructor's choice

CONDITIONING PHASE

(A set)

Knee-high jog with jog press

Run tires with jog press in front

Kick side to side

Jumping jacks

Cross-country ski and jumping jacks, alternate

Interval high-intensity phase: mini ski, faster

Interval active recovery phase: cross-country ski

Kick forward

(B set)

Knee-high jog, push forward, travel backward and forward

Knee-high jog with crawl stroke, travel backward and forward

Run tires with reverse breaststroke, travel backward and forward

Run tires with breaststroke, travel backward and forward

Kick side to side, travel backward and forward

Jumping jacks, travel backward and forward

Cross-country ski and jumping jacks, alternate

Interval high-intensity phase: cross-country ski, neutral position, full ROM

Interval active recovery phase: cross-country ski

Kick forward

(C set)
Knee-high jog with arm medley

(D set)
Knee-high jog, travel sideways

Leap sideways (low impact option: crab walk sideways)

Kick side to side, travel sideways

Jumping jacks, travel sideways

Cross-country ski and jumping jacks, alternate

Interval high-intensity phase: cross-country ski, suspended

Interval active recovery phase: cross-country ski, neutral position

Kick forward

(E set)
Crossover knees

In in, out out

Side kick (karate)

Jacks tuck

Cross-country ski and jumping jacks, alternate

Interval high-intensity phase: cross-country ski with power

Interval active recovery phase: cross-country ski

Kick forward

COOL-DOWN
Knee-high jog with jog press

Run tires with jog press in front

Kick side to side

Jumping jacks

(Straddle noodle)

Bicycle with reverse breaststroke and no hands, travel backward and forward

Seated leg press with paddle pull, travel backward and forward

Seated kick with reverse breaststroke and breaststroke, travel backward and forward

Seated jacks, travel backward and forward

(Stand on noodle)

Jumping jacks with one foot on noodle

Cross-country ski with one foot on noodle

(Kneel on noodle)

Kneel on noodle and balance

Travel backward with reverse breaststroke and forward with breaststroke

Stretch: hip flexors, gastrocnemius, hamstrings, outer thigh, lower back, shoulders

▶ **Shallow-Water Lesson Plan 29**

INTERVALS WITH SPEED

CLASS OBJECTIVE
Cardiorespiratory fitness

EQUIPMENT
None

TEACHING TIP
There are many ways to do intervals. One option is to apply one way of increasing intensity to different exercises in each set of block choreography. If you increase intensity with speed, encourage your participants not to lose their range of motion and make the move smaller. For the arm medley, choose any upper-body moves you like.

WARM-UP
Instructor's choice

CONDITIONING PHASE
(A set)
Rocking horse

Kick forward, travel backward and forward

High kick

Ankle touch, feet wide apart

Hopscotch, feet wide apart

Knee-high jog with unison push forward, travel backward and forward

Knee-high jog with standing row, travel backward and forward

Crossover knees

Interval high-intensity phase: knee-high jog, faster
Interval active recovery phase: knee-high jog

(B set)
Rocking horse with front kick
Kick forward, travel backward and forward
High kick
Ankle touch, feet close together
Hopscotch, feet close together
Cross-country ski, travel backward and forward
Cross-country ski with unison arm swing, travel backward and forward
Mini ski
Interval high-intensity phase: cross-country ski, faster
Interval active recovery phase: cross-country ski

(C set)
Knee-high jog with arm medley

(D set)
Rocking horse with shoulder blade squeeze
Kick forward, travel backward and forward
High kick
Ankle touch and hopscotch, alternate
Jumping jacks, travel backward and forward
Jumping jacks, clap hands, travel backward and forward
Mini jacks
Interval high-intensity phase: jumping jacks, faster
Interval active recovery phase: jumping jacks

(E set)
Knee lift and lunge
Kick forward, travel backward and forward
High kick
Ankle touch, one ankle only and hopscotch, one heel only; alternate
Jump backward and sprint, travel in a zigzag
Bicycle, small circles, suspended
Interval high-intensity phase: bicycle, faster, suspended
Interval active recovery phase: bicycle, suspended

COOL-DOWN
Pelvic tilt, standing
Side crunch, standing

Crunch, lunge position
Lower-body twist
Stand on one foot and extend leg, hands up
Fall forward, tuck and stand
Side fall, tuck and stand
Stretch: hamstrings, outer thigh, inner thigh, quadriceps, latissimus dorsi, shoulders

▶ **Shallow-Water Lesson Plan 30**

INTERVALS WITH ROM

CLASS OBJECTIVE
Cardiorespiratory fitness

EQUIPMENT
Noodles

TEACHING TIP
When you increase intensity by increasing range of motion, encourage participants to go to their personal full range of motion, even if theirs is different from those of others in the class. For the arm medley, choose any upper-body moves you like.

WARM-UP
Instructor's choice

CONDITIONING PHASE
(A set)
Rocking horse R and kick side to side
Rocking horse L and kick side to side
Run tires, travel backward and forward
Sprint
Kick forward, travel backward and forward
Kick forward with crossovers
Kick forward, doubles
Interval high-intensity phase: high kick
Interval active recovery phase: kick forward

(B set)
Rocking horse R and kick side to side
Rocking horse L and kick side to side
Run tires, travel sideways
Sprint
Jumping jacks, travel sideways
Jumping jacks, palms touch in front and in back
Jumping jacks, doubles

Interval high-intensity phase: jacks cross, full ROM
Interval active recovery phase: jumping jacks

(C set)
Rocking horse R and kick side to side
Rocking horse L and kick side to side
Run tires, travel backward and forward
Sprint
Cross-country ski, travel backward and forward
Cross-country ski with forearm press, side to side
Cross-country ski, doubles
Interval high-intensity phase: cross-country ski, full ROM
Interval active recovery phase: cross-country ski

(D set)
Knee-high jog with arm medley

COOL-DOWN
Rocking horse R and kick side to side
Rocking horse L and kick side to side
Run tires
(Straddle noodle)
Seated leg press, travel backward
Bicycle, no hands, travel forward
Seated jacks, travel backward and forward
Seated jacks, open and close doors
(Noodle behind shoulders)
Seated triple crossover
Seated jacks cross, full ROM
Hip curl, L position
Crunch, V position
Side-to-side extension, R leg only
Side-to-side extension, L leg only
Stretch: gastrocnemius, hip flexors, quadriceps, hamstrings, inner thigh, shoulders

▶ Shallow-Water Lesson Plan 31

INTERVALS WITH SUSPENDED MOVES

CLASS OBJECTIVES
Cardiorespiratory fitness and muscular strength and endurance

EQUIPMENT
Dumbbells (optional) and noodles

TEACHING TIP
If dumbbells are unavailable, ask your participants to push hard against the water in the lunge position at the beginning of the cool-down. If dumbbells are available, holding them in the hands with a noodle behind the shoulders adds extra stability to the side-lying exercises.

WARM-UP
Knee-high jog with jog press
Knee-high jog with unison jog press
Rocking horse
Cross-country ski
Kick forward with arm swing
Kick forward, push forward
Straddle jog with paddlewheel
Straddle jog with scull

CONDITIONING PHASE
(A set)
Skate kick
Ankle touch
High kick
Knee lift and lunge
Knee-high jog with shoulder blade squeeze
Knee-high jog, palms touch in back
Knee-high jog with triceps extension
Knee-high jog, one knee only, travel sideways
R knee lift, L kick forward, and repeat other side
Interval high-intensity phase: bicycle, suspended
Interval active recovery phase: knee-high jog, neutral position
Knee-high jog

(B set)
Skate kick
Ankle touch
High kick
Knee lift and lunge
Cross-country ski, clap hands
Cross-country ski with lat pull-down
Cross-country ski with alternating arm curl
Cross-country ski, travel sideways
Tuck ski

Interval high-intensity phase: cross-country ski, suspended

Interval active recovery phase: cross-country ski, neutral position

Cross-country ski

(C set)

Skate kick

Ankle touch

High kick

Knee lift and lunge

Kick forward with shoulder blade squeeze

Kick forward, palms touch in back

Kick forward with triceps extension

Kick forward, travel sideways

Chorus line kick

Interval high-intensity phase: kick forward, suspended

Interval active recovery phase: kick forward, neutral position

Kick forward

(D set)

Skate kick

Ankle touch

High kick

Knee lift and lunge

Straddle jog, clap hands

Straddle jog, palms touch in front

Straddle jog with arm curl

Straddle jog, travel sideways

Frog jump (low-impact option: neutral position)

Interval high-intensity phase: frog jump, suspended

Interval active recovery phase: straddle jog, neutral position

Straddle jog

COOL-DOWN

(Dumbbells in hands)

Shoulder blade squeeze (lunge position)

Dumbbells touch in back (lunge position)

Triceps extension (lunge position)

(Noodle behind shoulders and dumbbells in hands)

Bicycle, side-lying

Cross-country ski, side-lying

Flutter kick, side-lying

(Noodle in hands)

Side-to-side extension

Abdominal pike and spine extension

Stretch: shoulders, upper back, latissimus dorsi, triceps, hip flexors, hamstrings

▶ **Shallow-Water Lesson Plan 32**

INTERVALS WITH POWER

CLASS OBJECTIVE

Cardiorespiratory fitness

EQUIPMENT

Noodles

TEACHING TIP

It is sometimes difficult to teach adding power to a move. Use as many power words as you can think of, such as *force, effort, energy, intensity, make waves, might, use your muscles, push hard, strength, vigor,* and *high voltage.* It may also help to get in the water with your class and demonstrate.

WARM-UP

Jumping jacks

Jumping jacks, squat

Jacks tuck

Tuck ski

Cross-country ski

Rocking horse

Knee-high jog

Heel jog

Kick forward with reverse breaststroke and breaststroke, travel backward and forward

Jump backward and leap forward (low-impact option: jump backward and sprint forward)

CONDITIONING PHASE

(A set)

One leg kicks side

Jumping jacks, travel backward and forward

Jacks cross

Interval high-intensity phase: jumping jacks with power

Interval active recovery phase: jumping jacks

Kick forward with reverse breaststroke and breaststroke with power, travel backward and forward

Jump backward and leap forward (low-impact option: jump backward and sprint forward)

(B set)

One leg kicks forward and back

Cross-country ski, travel backward and forward

Cross-country ski, corner to corner

Interval high-intensity phase: cross-country ski with power

Interval active recovery phase: cross-country ski

Kick forward with reverse breaststroke with power and breaststroke, travel backward and forward

Jump backward and leap forward (low-impact option: jump backward and sprint forward)

(C set)

Knee-high jog, one knee only, travel sideways

Knee-high jog with double-arm press-down, travel backward and forward

Ankle touch

Interval high-intensity phase: steep climb

Interval active recovery phase: knee-high jog

Kick forward with breaststroke with power and reverse breaststroke, travel backward and forward

Jump backward and leap forward (low-impact option: jump backward and sprint forward)

(D set)

Heel jog, one heel only, travel sideways

Heel jog with forearm press, travel backward and forward

Hopscotch

Interval high-intensity phase: kick forward, suspended, with power; emphasize hamstrings

Interval active recovery phase: kick forward, neutral position

Kick forward with breaststroke and reverse breaststroke with power, travel backward and forward

Jump backward and leap forward (low-impact option: jump backward and sprint forward)

(E set) (Straddle noodle)

Seated kick with reverse breaststroke and breaststroke, travel backward and forward

Seated reverse breaststroke and breaststroke, travel backward and forward

Bicycle, one leg only

Bicycle with unison arm swing, travel backward and forward

Bicycle, tandem

Interval high-intensity phase: bicycle, climb a hill

Interval active recovery phase: bicycle

COOL-DOWN

Seated kick with reverse breaststroke and breaststroke, travel backward and forward

Seated reverse breaststroke and breaststroke, travel backward and forward

(Noodle in hands)

Diamond fall forward, tuck and stand

Side fall, tuck and stand

Abdominal pike and spine extension with legs in a diamond position

(Kneel on noodle)

Kneel on noodle and balance

Travel sideways with sidestroke

Stretch: hip flexors, quadriceps, hamstrings, outer thigh, upper back, pectorals

▶ Shallow-Water Lesson Plan 33

INTERVALS WITH SPEED AND SUSPENDED MOVES

CLASS OBJECTIVE

Cardiorespiratory fitness

EQUIPMENT

Noodles

TEACHING TIP

To add variety and challenge to your interval training, experiment with different ways of increasing intensity, using several different exercises. This lesson plan uses speed and suspended moves to increase intensity with knee-high jog, kick forward, cross-country ski, and run tires.

WARM-UP

Instructor's choice

CONDITIONING PHASE

(A set)

Kick forward

Jumping jacks

Heel jog

Skate kick

Knee-high jog, travel backward and forward

Interval high-intensity phase: knee-high jog, faster

Interval active recovery phase: knee-high jog

Interval high-intensity phase: bicycle, suspended

Interval active recovery phase: knee-high jog

Interval high-intensity phase: sprint

Interval active recovery phase: knee-high jog

Knee-high jog with breaststroke 4× and reverse breaststroke 4×, alternate

Breaststroke and reverse breaststroke, alternate (lunge position)

(B set)

Kick forward, travel backward and forward

Jumping jacks, travel sideways

Heel jog, travel backward and forward

Skate kick, travel backward and forward

Small kick, travel backward and forward

Interval high-intensity phase: jump flutter (low-impact option: small kick, faster)

Interval active recovery phase: kick forward

Interval high-intensity phase: kick forward, suspended

Interval active recovery phase: kick forward

Interval high-intensity phase: kick forward, faster

Interval active recovery phase: kick forward

Knee-high jog with lat pull-down

Knee-high jog with double-arm press-down

Lat pull-down and double-arm press-down, alternate (lunge position)

(C set)

High kick, travel backward and forward

Jumping jacks, clap hands, travel backward and forward

Skip rope, travel backward and forward

Knee lift and lunge

Cross-country ski, travel backward and forward

Interval high-intensity phase: mini ski, faster

Interval active recovery phase: cross-country ski

Interval high-intensity phase: cross-country ski, suspended

Interval active recovery phase: cross-country ski

Interval high-intensity phase: cross-country ski, faster

Interval active recovery phase: cross-country ski

Knee-high jog with arm curl

Knee-high jog with triceps extension

Arm curl, palms face direction of motion (lunge position)

(D set)

Kick forward, neutral position

Jumping jacks, neutral position

Rocking horse

In-line skate

Run tires, travel backward and forward

Interval high-intensity phase: run tires, faster

Interval active recovery phase: run tires

Interval high-intensity phase: run tires, suspended

Interval active recovery phase: run tires

Interval high-intensity phase: run tires, faster, travel forward

Interval active recovery phase: run tires

Knee-high jog with forearm press

Forearm press, side to side (lunge position)

COOL-DOWN

(Noodle behind shoulders)

Seated jacks

Seated mini cross

Seated triple crossover

Crunch, V position

Eight short crunches and two long crunches

Stretch: hamstrings, quadriceps, hip flexors, pectorals, latissimus dorsi, triceps, shoulders

▶ **Shallow-Water Lesson Plan 34**

INTERVALS WITH SUSPENDED MOVES AND POWER

CLASS OBJECTIVE
Cardiorespiratory fitness

EQUIPMENT
Noodles

TEACHING TIP
The side fall and the fall forward both work the core stabilizers, but they also train participants how to recover from a fall in the water.

WARM-UP
Instructor's choice

CONDITIONING PHASE
(A set)
Kick forward, neutral position with scull
Kick forward, palms touch in back
Crossover knees
Ankle touch
Knee-high jog with crossovers
Knee-high jog, clap hands, travel backward
Sprint, travel in a zigzag
Cross-country ski, travel backward and forward
Interval high-intensity phase: cross-country ski, suspended
Interval active recovery phase: cross-country ski, neutral position
Interval high-intensity phase: bicycle, suspended
Interval active recovery phase: tuck ski

(B set)
Kick forward, neutral position, travel backward and forward
Kick forward, travel backward and forward
Crossover knees
Ankle touch, doubles
Knee-high jog with double-arm lift
Knee-high jog with double-arm press-down, travel backward
Sprint, travel in a zigzag
Cross-country ski, travel sideways

Interval high-intensity phase: cross-country ski with power
Interval active recovery phase: cross-country ski
Interval high-intensity phase: steep climb
Interval active recovery phase: knee-high jog

(C set)
Kick forward, suspended
One leg kicks forward
Crossover knees
Ankle touch, one ankle only
Knee-high jog, open and close doors
Knee-high jog with breaststroke, travel backward
Sprint, travel in a zigzag
Cross-country ski, travel backward and forward
Interval high-intensity phase: cross-country ski, suspended
Interval active recovery phase: cross-country ski, neutral position
Interval high-intensity phase: bicycle, suspended
Interval active recovery phase: tuck ski

(D set)
Mermaid, suspended
Kick forward, low to high, 4×
Crossover knees
Ankle touch with double arms
Knee-high jog with forearm press
Knee-high jog, push forward, travel backward
Sprint, travel in a zigzag
Cross-country ski, travel sideways
Interval high-intensity phase: cross-country ski with power
Interval active recovery phase: cross-country ski
Interval high-intensity phase: steep climb
Interval active recovery phase: knee-high jog

COOL-DOWN
(Noodle behind shoulders)
Cross-country ski, side-lying, travel
Seated flutter kick
Knee-high jog, side-lying, travel
Seated high kick
Tuck ski together, side-lying, travel
Flutter kick up to L position and down to the floor

Bicycle, side-lying, travel

Hip curl from a kneeling position

Side-to-side extension with legs in a diamond position (Noodle in hands)

Abdominal pike and spine extension with legs in a diamond position

Side fall, tuck and stand on one foot

Fall forward, tuck and stand on one foot

Stretch: gastrocnemius, hip flexors, quadriceps, hamstrings, shoulders, pectorals

▶ Shallow-Water Lesson Plan 35

INTERVALS WITH SPEED, ROM, AND SUSPENDED MOVES

CLASS OBJECTIVE
Cardiorespiratory fitness

EQUIPMENT
Noodles

TEACHING TIP
Try organizing two exercises in a pyramid, as follows: a 8×, b 8×, a 4×, b 4×, a 2×, b 2×, a, b. You can also reverse the order, beginning with "a" and "b" alternating and working up to eight times. For the arm medley, choose any upper-body moves you like.

WARM-UP
Knee-high jog with jog press

Knee-high jog, palms touch in back

Straddle jog with shoulder blade squeeze

Heel jog with triceps extension

Knee-high jog with scull

Knee-high jog, scull arms down, travel backward and forward

Knee-high jog, travel sideways

CONDITIONING PHASE
(A set)

Kick forward

Kick side to side, travel backward and forward

Side quad kick, travel sideways

Kick to the corners

Kick forward and kick to the corners, pyramid (see teaching tip for this lesson plan)

Interval high-intensity phase: kick forward, faster

Interval active recovery phase: kick forward

Interval high-intensity phase: high kick

Interval active recovery phase: kick and lunge

Interval high-intensity phase: kick forward, suspended

Interval active recovery phase: front kick (karate)

Kick forward

(B set)

Cross-country ski

Jumping jacks, clap hands, travel backward and forward

Jumping jacks, squat, travel sideways

Jumping jacks

Cross-country ski and jumping jacks, pyramid

Interval high-intensity phase: cross-country ski, faster

Interval active recovery phase: cross-country ski

Interval high-intensity phase: cross-country ski, neutral position, full ROM

Interval active recovery phase: tuck ski

Interval high-intensity phase: cross-country ski, suspended

Interval active recovery phase: tuck ski, corner to corner

Cross-country ski

(C set)

Knee-high jog with arm medley

(D set)

Knee-high jog

Run tires, travel backward and forward

Rocking horse to the side, travel sideways

Run tires

Knee-high jog and run tires, pyramid

Interval high-intensity phase: knee-high jog, faster

Interval active recovery phase: knee-high jog

Interval high-intensity phase: leap forward (low-impact option: sprint)

Interval active recovery phase: knee lift and lunge

Interval high-intensity phase: bicycle, suspended

Interval active recovery phase: chorus line kick

Knee-high jog

COOL-DOWN

(Noodle behind shoulders)

Flutter kick, side-lying, travel

Cross-country ski, side-lying, travel

Bicycle, side-lying, travel

(Noodle in hands)

Side-to-side extension

Abdominal pike and spine extension

Extension forward, R, back, L, and reverse

Stretch: inner thigh, outer thigh, hamstrings, quadriceps, obliques, shoulders, triceps

▶ Shallow-Water Lesson Plan 36

INTERVALS WITH SPEED, ROM, SUSPENDED MOVES, AND POWER

CLASS OBJECTIVE

Cardiorespiratory fitness

EQUIPMENT

Noodles

TEACHING TIP

Sometimes participants are more likely to drink water if you offer them water breaks. Don't forget to drink water yourself!

WARM-UP

Knee-high jog with jog press

Walk backward and forward 2×

Step sideways 2×

Walk 4×, jog 8×

CONDITIONING PHASE

(A set)

One leg kicks forward and back

Ankle touch

Hopscotch

Heel jog with shoulder blade squeeze

Cross-country ski, corner to corner

Jumping jacks, clap hands, travel backward and forward

Knee-high jog with breaststroke, travel backward and forward

Interval high-intensity phase: knee-high jog, faster

Interval active recovery phase: knee-high jog

Interval high-intensity phase: jump flutter (low-impact option: mini ski, faster)

Interval active recovery phase: knee-high jog

Interval high-intensity phase: knee-high jog, faster

Interval active recovery phase: knee-high jog

(B set)

One leg kicks forward and back

Ankle touch with double arms

Hopscotch

Heel jog with shoulder blade squeeze

Cross-country ski with unison arm swing

Jumping jacks, travel sideways

Knee-high jog with windshield wiper arms, travel backward and forward

Interval high-intensity phase: high kick

Interval active recovery phase: kick forward

Interval high-intensity phase: cross-country ski, full ROM

Interval active recovery phase: kick forward

Interval high-intensity phase: high kick

Interval active recovery phase: kick forward

(C set)

One leg kicks forward and back

Ankle touch with double arms

Hopscotch, one heel only

Heel jog with shoulder blade squeeze

Cross-country ski, push forward

Jumping jacks with arm curl, travel backward and forward

Knee-high jog with triceps extension, travel backward and forward

Interval high-intensity phase: jumping jacks, suspended

Interval active recovery phase: kick forward, neutral position

Interval high-intensity phase: bicycle, faster, suspended

Interval active recovery phase: kick forward, neutral position

Interval high-intensity phase: jumping jacks, suspended

Interval active recovery phase: kick forward, neutral position

(D set)

One leg kicks forward and back

Ankle touch with double arms

Hopscotch, doubles

Heel jog with shoulder blade squeeze

Cross-country ski with forearm press, side to side

Jumping jacks, palms touch in back, travel backward and forward

Knee-high jog with forearm press, travel backward and forward

Interval high-intensity phase: steep climb

Interval active recovery phase: knee-high jog

Interval high-intensity phase: cross-country ski with power

Interval active recovery phase: knee-high jog

Interval high-intensity phase: steep climb

Interval active recovery phase: knee-high jog

COOL-DOWN:

Walk 4×, jog 8×

Walk backward and forward

Step sideways

(Noodle behind shoulders)

Side-to-side extension

Bicycle, side-lying, in a circle

Hip curl, V position

Crunch, V position

V-sit

Stretch: pectorals, upper back, shoulders, hip flexors, hamstrings, quadriceps, outer thigh

PART II

DEEP-WATER EXERCISE

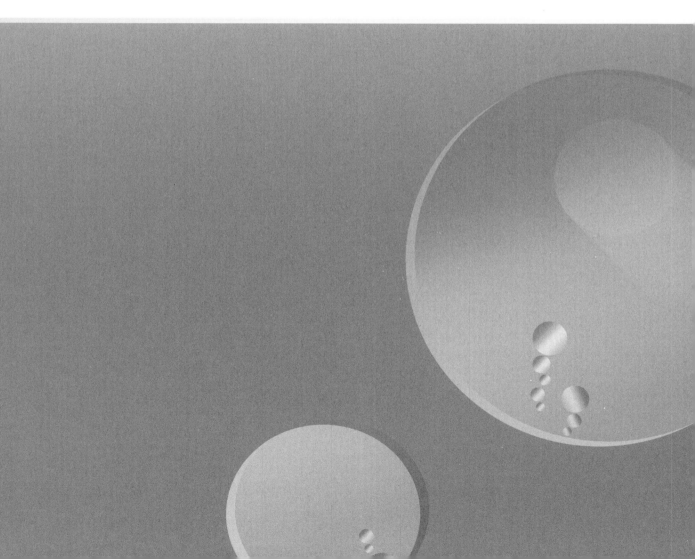

CHAPTER 4

Introduction to Deep-Water Exercise

If you have an opportunity to teach a deep-water class, it is important to understand the differences between shallow-water and deep-water exercise. The most obvious difference, of course, is that in shallow-water exercise, participants can stand on the bottom of the pool, whereas deep-water exercise takes place in water that is over participants' heads. Therefore, they need to wear some kind of flotation device. The most common flotation device is a deep-water belt, but cuffs for the upper arms and cuffs for the ankles are also available.

Deep-water belts come in a variety of styles and sizes. Correct fit depends on the size and shape of the participant. Have your participants float upright in the water with their arms down at their sides. A person whose shoulders are several inches above the water needs a belt with less buoyancy. A person whose chin is touching the water needs a belt with more buoyancy. Those who tend to pitch forward need belts with less buoyancy in back, and those who tend to pitch backward need a belt with less buoyancy in front. The solution in either case may be to fasten the belt in the back instead of in the front or to try a different style of belt (AEA, 2006).

A second difference between shallow-water and deep-water exercise has to do with the fact that our bodies normally receive information about our posture through contact with the ground (AEA, 2006). With no floor to stand on in deep water, the working environment is unstable. Participants may experience a lack of balance and coordination. They have to learn how to balance using their center of buoyancy, which is located in the chest, instead of their center of gravity, which is located in the pelvic area (Stuart, 2009). Often participants let their legs float up as if they were sitting in a chair, or they curl their chests forward. Neutral posture is important to minimize stress on the spine, and it is the safest position for preventing injury when the arms and legs are working (see figure 4.1; AEA, 2006). In neutral posture, the spine is aligned in its natural curves. Dropping the chin forward, rounding the shoulders, flexing forward at the waist, and twisting to one side, all take the spine out of neutral. To achieve neutral posture in deep water, participants must engage the muscles of the core (AEA, 2006). This takes some practice. You will need to give your participants frequent cues for good posture,

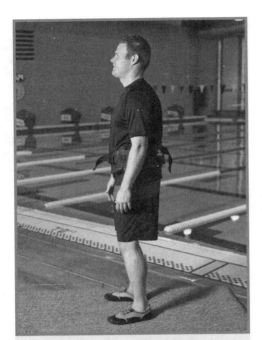

FIGURE 4.1 **Neutral posture is the safest position for preventing injury when the arms and legs are working in water fitness exercises.**

such as: *Head over shoulders, shoulders over hips, and feet under you.* Ask them to elongate their bodies and return to their vertical alignment with each repetition of an exercise. It is also helpful to teach them how to scull, or sweep the hands outward with the thumbs angled down and inward with the thumbs angled up, which will help them stabilize.

Buoyancy constitutes another important difference between deep-water and shallow-water exercise. Buoyancy reduces the stress on the joints in deep water, even more than in shallow water, making deep-water exercise ideal for people with hip, knee, or foot issues. It also decreases the compressive load on the spine, which makes it a good choice for those with low back problems, provided they have enough core strength to maintain neutral alignment (AEA, 2006).

The working positions of rebounding, neutral (with the hips and knees flexed and the shoulders at the surface of the water), and suspended do not apply to deep water. However, in deep water participants can lean diagonally to the side with some of the exercises. They can add elevation by pulling the arms and legs together forcefully, or use a scull to lift the shoulders out of the water. They can raise the arms out of the water to make the body sink and force the legs to work harder. Raising the arms overhead, however, stimulates the pressor response and raises the heart rate. Limit the length of time your participants work with the hands overhead to 15 to 30 seconds, or cue raising the hands to just above the ears. Participants with high blood pressure should not raise their hands above their heads (YMCA, 2000). You can have participants perform moves side lying, seated in an L position, or seated in a dining room chair position without having to get out a noodle, giving you the freedom to insert these moves into your lesson plan whenever you wish to decrease intensity. Be aware that diagonal and side-lying moves are difficult to perform with ankle cuffs. If your participants are using this type of flotation device, avoid using these positions in your lesson plans.

The need for flotation devices, the unstable environment, the elimination of stress on the joints, and the deep-water working positions differentiate deep-water exercise from shallow-water exercise. Nevertheless, designing deep-water classes is similar to designing shallow-water classes.

PREPARING YOUR CLASS

You need to plan ahead for your deep-water classes just as you do for your shallow-water classes. Begin by determining your class objective, which can either be cardiorespiratory fitness or muscular strength and endurance. See chapter 1 for information on these objectives. As with shallow-water classes, you need to include a warm-up, a conditioning phase, and a cool-down in every class.

WARM-UP PHASE

The warm-up phase in a deep-water class must accomplish two things. Participants not only have to make a body temperature adjustment to the colder temperature of the water, as in a shallow-water class, but they also have to adjust to the unstable environment in deep water. An upright posture is important to maintain the spine in neutral alignment so that all the exercises can be performed safely. Good posture, however, is not automatic in deep water. Begin the warm-up with a vigorous, short-lever move, such as a knee-high jog, while offering postural cues to help participants achieve neutral alignment. Teach them how to scull, which will help them stabilize. As they begin to feel more comfortable, you can begin to increase their heart rates in preparation for the workout. The entire warm-up should take between 5 and 10 minutes.

One way to warm up is to jog in place for two to three minutes; then scull with other short-lever leg moves such as a straddle jog, flutter kick, or Cossack kick. Add moves that recruit the core, such as a jacks tuck or a seated kick, to help participants maintain balance and alignment (Stuart, 2009). Finally, add longer-lever moves. If your participants are more experienced, they can warm up by jogging with various arm moves. Have them perform a knee-high jog, a straddle jog, and a heel jog to use different leg muscles as they warm up the upper body. You can use the warm-up to introduce moves that may be new to them. Begin with a knee-high jog and sculling, and then introduce the new moves at half speed, increasing to regular water tempo as the participants catch on to the moves. The following two sample warm-ups will get you started.

FIVE-MINUTE WARM-UP

Knee-high jog with jog press (1 min.)

Knee-high jog with scull (30 secs.)

Straddle jog with scull (30 secs.)

Run tires with scull (30 secs.)

Cossack kick (30 secs.)

Seated kick with scull (30 secs.)

Jacks tuck (30 secs.)

Tuck ski (30 secs.)

Bicycle with scull (30 secs.)

TEN-MINUTE WARM-UP

Knee-high jog with jog press (1 min.)

Knee-high jog with shoulder blade squeeze (1 min.)

Straddle jog, palms touch in front (1 min.)

Straddle jog, palms touch in back (1 min.)

Cossack kick (30 secs.)

Ankle touch (30 secs.)

Hopscotch (30 secs.)

Jumping jacks (30 secs.)

Jacks tuck (30 secs.)

Tuck ski (30 secs.)

Cross-country ski, knees bent 90 degrees (30 secs.)

Cross-country ski (30 secs.)

Bicycle (30 secs.)

Bicycle, scull in front, travel backward (45 secs.)

Bicycle, scull arms down, travel forward (45 secs.)

By the end of the warm-up, the water will feel comfortable or even slightly warm to your participants, they will be breathing a bit harder, and their muscles will be ready for the increased intensity of the conditioning phase.

CONDITIONING PHASE

The conditioning phase is the main section of your class, and it takes up the major portion of your class time. Your participants are there for a workout to maintain or improve their current level of physical fitness. Two of the components of physical fitness are cardiorespiratory endurance, and muscular strength and endurance (USWFA, 2007). The American College of Sports Medicine has made recommendations that you will want to keep in mind when you design the conditioning phase of your lesson plan to focus on one or both of these components. See chapter 1 for information about the American College of Sports Medicine's recommendations for physical activity.

Conditioning Phase: Cardiorespiratory Fitness

Working on cardiorespiratory fitness in a deep-water class presents certain challenges. Because the lungs are completely submerged, breathing may feel more difficult. This gives participants the impression that they are working harder than they actually are. Encourage them to breathe deeply. They will learn to adjust to this sensation over time (YMCA, 2000). Ninety percent of the body is submerged in deep-water exercise. The arms and legs must work against the resistance of the water, and the muscles may accumulate lactic acid and become fatigued. This contributes to an increased perception of work (AEA, 2006). Your participants will need some experience before they can effectively use Borg's rating of perceived exertion scale. A heart rate monitor can be a useful aid for judging working intensity in deep water. A heart rate chart such as the one in table 4.1 can give them an idea of what their target heart rates should be.

This heart rate chart in table 4.1 takes into account the fact that the human heart has an estimate of 17 beats per minute fewer in deep water than on land. Heart rates in deep water are lower than heart rates in shallow water, although the exercise intensity is the same as on land. This may be because a greater percentage of the body is submerged in deep water (AEA, 2006). Certain medications and the fitness level of the participant also affect heart rate. Therefore, heart rate charts cannot be accurate for everyone, and should be used only to establish general guidelines.

Maximum heart rate is determined by using the formula 220 minus age (USWFA, 2007). For cardiorespiratory fitness, a heart rate of between 60 and 80 percent of maximum heart rate is considered appropriate (AEA, 2006). This range is referred to as the target heart rate (USWFA, 2007). Participants who want to do moderately intense cardio work, work out in the lower level of the target heart rate, and those who want to do vigorously intense cardio work, work out in the upper level of the target heart rate.

Target heart rates are achieved by working large-muscle groups continuously and rhythmically. The two options for meeting the objective of training for car-

TABLE 4.1

Target Heart Rates in Deep Water

Formula: [(220 − age) × % intensity] − 17

Age	% INTENSITY						
	55%	60%	65%	70%	75%	80%	85%
25	90	100	110	120	129	139	149
30	88	97	107	116	126	135	145
35	85	94	103	113	122	131	140
40	82	91	100	109	118	127	136
45	79	88	97	106	114	123	132
50	77	85	94	102	111	119	128
55	74	82	90	99	107	115	123
60	71	79	87	95	103	111	119
65	68	76	84	92	99	107	115
70	66	73	81	88	96	103	111
75	63	70	77	85	92	99	106
80	60	67	74	81	88	95	102

diorespiratory fitness are a continuous training format and an interval training format.

Continuous Training Format. In continuous training, you bring your participants up to their target heart rates and have them remain there for the duration of the conditioning phase. The conditioning phase should last at least 30 minutes to meet the American College of Sports Medicine's recommendations for moderate physical activity (ACSM, 2007). Your class should include exercises that use large-muscle groups continuously and rhythmically. Save many of your seated and side-lying moves as well as abdominal and balance exercises for the cool-down portion of your class because they will bring the heart rate down. The best way to see if your exercise selection is appropriate is to practice the moves ahead of time wearing a heart rate monitor.

Interval Training Format. In interval training, you bring your participants up to the lower or midlevel of their target heart rates. Then you periodically increase the intensity so that their heart rates climb into the upper level of their target heart rates for a short time before decreasing the intensity to let the heart rates go back into the mid- or lower level. Interval training is great for improving cardiorespiratory fitness. Interval training, with its periods of active recovery when intensity is decreased, allows for the removal of lactic acid and is a good way to overcome the fatigue associated with working in deep water (AEA, 2006). The two things you need to know to lead an interval class are how to increase and decrease intensity, and how long to work in the upper level of the target heart rate.

Following are five factors you can address to increase intensity in deep water:

1. Speed
2. Range of motion
3. Elevation
4. Power
5. Travel

Increasing speed results in performing the move faster without compromising range of motion. You need to be aware that resistance in water is three-dimensional, and it increases exponentially with force. The harder you push against the water, the harder it pushes back. This exaggerated action/reaction effect makes it difficult to gain sufficient speed to achieve desired intensity levels in deep water (YMCA, 2000). Often participants go faster but make the move smaller. If you have beginners, it may be best to use a different way to increase intensity until they become more experienced. Increasing range of motion involves performing exercises with long levers (arms and legs slightly flexed) through their full range of motion. With elevation, participants either use a scull to lift the shoulders out of the water while working the legs very hard, or pull the arms and legs together forcefully enough to lift the shoulders out of the water. Increasing power is about pushing harder against the resistance of the water.

Travel involves moving through the water from one part of the pool to another. Travel in deep water requires upper-body strength, but it is also a learned skill. Participants have to know when to push or pull hard against the water and when to slice to get the body moving in the desired direction. They can travel forward, backward, or sideways. It's a good idea to have them pause and check for neutral posture before changing directions when traveling in deep water. This is especially important if they are traveling in the diagonal position. They should return to vertical and check their alignment before they lean diagonally in the opposite direction.

With practice and skill, your participants will be able to achieve very high levels of intensity in deep-water exercise (AEA, 2006). In the lesson plans in this book, the exercises used to bring the heart rate up during an interval session are labeled *interval high-intensity phase.*

To decrease intensity, your participants can slow down, decrease their range of motion, allow their shoulders to drop down from the elevated position, ease back on the power moves, or perform the exercise in place. In the lesson plans with intervals in this book, the exercises used to decrease heart rate following the high-intensity phase are labeled *interval active recovery phase.*

Timing the Intervals.   How long you work your class in the upper level of the target heart rate depends on the fitness levels of your participants. See chapter 1 for a discussion of the various options for timing the intervals.

Conditioning Phase: Muscular Strength and Endurance

To focus on muscular strength and endurance in deep water, you will use different strategies than you use in shallow water. It is not possible to stand in a lunge position while focusing on upper-body work, for example. Instead, participants will have to perform a stabilizing move such as a knee-high jog or a cross-country ski while moving their arms in coordination with their legs (YMCA, 2000). Ask your participants to push hard against the resistance of the water with their palms facing the direction of motion. The more force they use, the greater the resistance. To introduce strength training for the lower body, you can add force, or power, to leg moves.

Another option for focusing on muscular strength and endurance is to add equipment. Webbed gloves increase the resistance for the upper body, and some participants like to bring their own to class. Many facilities have noodles or foam dumbbells. Avoid doing an entire class with foam dumbbells, though, because that puts too much strain on the shoulder joint. Before you use any piece of equipment, make sure you know how to use it. The circuit format, which is a popular way to do muscular strength and endurance training in the water, works as well in deep water as it does in shallow. See chapter 1 for information about the various ways to teach a circuit class.

Core Strength Training. Deep water is all about core strength. Participants must continually contract the core muscles to maintain stability in deep water. But it is also possible to teach a class for more experienced participants that challenges core stability specifically (see Deep-Water Lesson Plan 9: Core Challenge). Asymmetrical moves such as moving one leg while keeping the other leg stationary make the postural muscles work harder. Avoid these kinds of moves if you have anyone in your class who will compromise body alignment trying to perform them.

Combining Cardiorespiratory Fitness and Strength Training. You can combine cardiorespiratory fitness and strength training by adding travel. Travel in deep water requires upper-body strength because there is no floor to push off from. Travel is also a way to increase intensity when you are working on cardiorespiratory fitness. By focusing on the muscles they are training, while traveling through water at maximum speed, participants are effectively working on cardiorespiratory fitness and muscular strength and endurance at the same time. You can also incorporate strength training into an interval class. Combine upper-body moves with aerobic exercises to bring your participants up to the lower or midlevel of their target heart rates. In this case, the overload for strength training comes from pushing hard against the water or from using webbed gloves.

Every 5 to 10 minutes during the conditioning phase, increase the intensity with speed, range of motion, elevation, power, or travel as described earlier so that the heart rate climbs into the upper level of the target heart rate for a short time before decreasing the intensity to let the heart rate go back into the mid- or lower level. It is a good idea to include exercises for the upper body in your cardio classes even when muscular strength and endurance is not your class objective. You can have participants do arm exercises while performing leg moves or add an arm medley with a knee-high jog.

Conditioning Phase: Choreography Options

Your lesson plan is a list of the exercises you plan to use in your class. Choreography is the way you organize those exercises to give them logic and flow and make them easy to remember. The four choreography strategies presented in this book are linear choreography, variations on a theme, add-on choreography, and block choreography. They are discussed more fully in chapter 1. The only difference to note when writing choreography for deep water is when using variations on a theme, in which two or three exercises are worked through multiple variations. You can add arm moves and increase speed. The leg moves across the body, the move combinations, and travel will be similar to shallow water, but the working positions will be different. Instead of using the neutral position, suspended moves, and rebounding, you will use the side-lying and seated positions, elevation, and hands up (if appropriate for your participants).

The conditioning phase is the most important part of your class, and you have many options! You can choose between the two class objectives of cardiorespiratory fitness and muscular strength and endurance, or you can combine both objectives into one class. If you choose to focus on cardiorespiratory fitness, you can use a continuous training format or an interval format. If you choose to focus on muscular strength and endurance, you can have participants overload the muscles without equipment by pushing hard against the resistance of the water, or you can have them use equipment. You can try a circuit format. Or you can combine the objectives of cardiorespiratory fitness and muscular strength and endurance in an interval class or by having participants travel. You can organize your lesson plans into four different choreography styles. With all these ideas, it is easy to keep your participants—and yourself—interested and challenged. Once you have completed your conditioning phase, it is time to begin the cool-down.

COOL-DOWN PHASE

The cool-down allows participants to slowly recover from the work they have done in the conditioning phase. If your last set ended with an interval, you should continue the active recovery exercise for a few minutes. Then you can begin to go into slower, lower-intensity movement. One way to do this is to repeat the warm-up, perhaps in reverse order. Another option is to include a set of toning exercises. These can be exercises for muscular strength, or they can be abdominal and core strength exercises.

Because flexibility is also important, finish your cool-down with at least five minutes of stretching. Participants can do static stretches for the major muscles they worked during the class, holding each stretch for 10 to 30 seconds. They should jog or bicycle for stability while they stretch the upper body, or stretch holding on to the wall. Dynamic stretching is also possible by moving the muscles slowly through their full range of motion.

MODIFYING YOUR LESSON PLAN FOR DIFFERENT POPULATIONS

You cannot assume that everyone in your class has the same fitness level that you have. Neither should you assume that just because your participants are older, they need a gentle workout. Observe your participants to see what they are capable of, and teach to those capabilities. Offer options for participants who want a higher intensity level as well as options for those who need a lower intensity level from the rest of the class. For example, you could teach a cross-country ski, and then give your participants the option to travel. Participants who need to work at a lower intensity can remain stationary and perform the move more slowly.

In general, older adults need a longer warm-up to allow time for their joints to warm up. Include movements that change direction to improve balance and coordination. Also include muscular strengthening and stretching exercises (AEA, 2006).

If your class includes men, use more callisthenic-type moves such as jumping jacks and cross-country ski. Keep your choreography simple, and have participants stay with a move for at least eight repetitions or longer before changing to another move. Men are often unwilling to participate in partner moves. Circuit classes and classes with muscular strength and endurance as their objective work well.

You may have participants in your class who have arthritis. Many people with mild to moderate arthritis do well in a regular fitness class. Participants with moderate to severe arthritis may be better served in an arthritis class. Contact the Arthritis Foundation to take their certification class if you wish to be involved in these types of classes. The Arthritis Foundation (www.arthritis.org) offers training for a deep-water arthritis class.

Cardiac patients, disabled people, and rehab patients need guidance from a doctor or a physical therapist. Working with athletes requires special training. Be sure you are qualified before taking on special populations that need skills beyond those taught in a typical certification class.

MUSIC

Your next step in preparing to teach your class is to decide whether you will use music. For more information on music and on U.S. copyright laws, see chapter 1. Because a greater range of motion can be achieved in deep water than in shallow water, choose music with a slightly slower tempo. Music that is 125 to 130 beats per minute works well for deep-water exercise, and with all of the deep-water choreography in this book.

TEACHING YOUR CLASS

Always arrive early to check out the pool before your class. What area of the pool will your participants be using? If you are using equipment, where is it located? If you are using music, where is the music player kept? Where are the locker rooms? Are there any tripping hazards between the locker room and the pool that you need to clear out of the way? Is the pool deck wet or slippery? Where will you stand when you teach your class? Remember that if you get in the pool to teach a deep-water class, your participants will not be able to see what you are doing. This will only work if your class has experience with your cues and experience in maintaining neutral posture. If you have beginners, it is better to teach from the deck where they will be able to see you and you will be able to see them. Don't forget to wear good, supportive water fitness shoes, and use a mat. It's a good feeling to know that you are prepared with your lesson plan and that your pool space is as safe as you can make it as you wait to greet your participants.

TROUBLESHOOTING

- **What should you do if one of your participants is afraid of water?** Fear of water is difficult to handle in deep water. Arm cuffs, if your facility has them, may offer more stability than a deep-water belt. You can also give the participant a set of foam dumbbells to hold. Tell her to keep them to the sides on the surface of the water, with a slight bend in her elbows and her shoulders relaxed. In this position she can perform the leg movements but not the upper-body movements. When she gains confidence, she can put the dumbbells aside and add the arm work. Do not allow her to hang from the wall with her back to the wall and her elbows on the deck because this has the potential of injuring her shoulder joints (AEA, 2006). After a few classes, she may begin to overcome her fear of water. If not, you may need to suggest that she try a shallow-water class instead.

■ **What should you do if one of your participants tips over during class and is unable to return to vertical?** If he is on his back, have him tuck his knees into his chest and bring his head and shoulders forward, while pulling his arms upward in front. If he has tipped forward, have him tuck his knees into his chest and press his arms down in front (AEA, 2006). If you have any participants who seem especially unbalanced in deep water, teach the entire class how to recover to vertical before such an incident occurs.

■ **What should you do if some of your participants are not achieving neutral alignment during the class?** First, check to see if their flotation belts fit properly. If their belts are causing them to pitch forward or backward, ask them to try using different belts or to fasten their belts in the back instead of the front. Sometimes, however, a participant may think she is using good form when she is not. Ask everyone to check and make sure their feet are under their bodies. Remind them that good alignment is necessary to perform the exercises safely. Because the abdominal and back muscles must contract to maintain proper alignment, it sometimes helps to tell participants that maintaining good posture will work their abs for the entire class period. You can also give everyone a set of dumbbells and have them hold them to the sides on the surface of the water with a slight bend in the elbows and the shoulders relaxed, and then ask them to perform various leg moves. This will often pull them into better alignment. Have them put the dumbbells down and perform the same moves adding arm movements and maintaining the same alignment. It takes practice to learn what neutral alignment feels like.

■ **What should you do if one of your participants wants to take your deep-water class without using a flotation device?** Some participants believe they will work harder if they don't use a flotation device. It is true that they are likely to become fatigued treading water for the entire class period, but that is not the same thing as getting a good workout. Explain that they will find themselves sinking when they are vertical, so they will lean forward. In this position they cannot properly work the core muscles; neither can they work all of the muscles of the upper body and legs. If they try to solve the problem by using handheld buoyant equipment for all or most of the class, they risk injuring their shoulder joints. If they lose their grip on the handheld buoyant equipment, they risk going underwater and may panic. Explain that for all of these reasons, you require all your participants to wear flotation equipment that attaches to the body (AEA, 2006).

■ **What should you do if your participants fill up your space in the pool and there is not enough room for traveling?** You can have them get in a circle around the perimeter of your area and travel toward the center of the circle and back, or they can travel clockwise or counterclockwise. Currents do not form in deep water as they do in shallow water. Chapter 1 has additional ideas for how to maximize traveling in a small space, as well as other troubleshooting tips.

PUTTING IT ALL TOGETHER

You now have some tools for teaching deep-water classes. Deep water is similar to shallow water in that you need a class objective—cardiorespiratory fitness, muscular strength and endurance, or both. Your deep-water class, like shallow-water classes, is also divided into three parts—the warm-up, the conditioning phase, and the cool-down. You now have some ideas for designing each part. You have strategies for how to increase and decrease intensity in deep water to help your participants work in their target heart rates. You can organize the exercises into logical patterns using linear choreography, variations on a theme, add-on choreography, and block choreography, just as you do in shallow water. You also have some suggestions for troubleshooting when the unexpected happens. Now you are ready for a look at the exercises and cueing tips in chapter 5.

REFERENCES

ACSM. (2007). *Physical Activity and Public Health Guidelines*. Retrieved August 20, 2009, from American College of Sports Medicine: www.acsm.org//AM/Template.cfm?Section = Home_Page.

AEA. (2006). *Aquatic Fitness Professional Manual*. Champaign, IL: Human Kinetics.

Stuart, C. (2009, October). Going Deep. *Aquatics International*, pp. 38-40.

USWFA. (2007). *National Water Fitness Instructors Manual*. Boynton Beach, FL: United States Water Fitness Association.

YMCA. (2000). *YMCA Water Fitness for Health*. Champaign, IL: Human Kinetics.

CHAPTER 5

Deep-Water Exercises and Cueing Tips

The list of deep-water exercises begins with exercises for cardiovascular fitness— jog, bicycle, kick, cross-country ski, jumping jacks, and variations of each. By adding power, most of the exercises can also be used to build muscular strength and endurance. This chapter also includes a section on using upper-body moves to assist travel. For further upper-body moves, see chapter 2. Although good form in deep-water exercise strengthens the core muscles, this chapter includes a section on additional strength training exercises for abdominals and obliques, followed by a list of more advanced exercises to challenge the core muscles.

Some of these exercise groups—jog; kick; and the exercises for the abdominals and obliques—are further divided into sub-groups, which are indicated by boldface type and italics for the title of the first exercise in each sub-group. The muscles used for each exercise and the variations are listed. At the end of each group and sub-group, the directions of travel are listed that are possible for that group of exercises, along with instructions for how to accomplish travel in that direction in deep water. The muscles used here will be the same for the stationary exercise in addition to the muscles used in any travel-assisting upper-body exercise you choose to include.

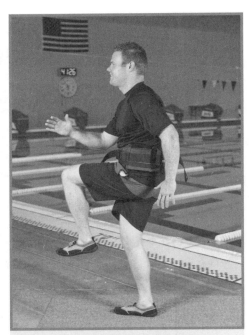

FIGURE 5.1 Knee-high jog: Jog with the knee coming up to hip level.

JOG

Knee-high jog (hip and knee flexion) (see figure 5.1); *muscles used:* hip flexors, hamstrings, quadriceps

▶ **CUEING TIP:** Bring the knee up to hip level; push the heels down toward the floor.

Knee-high jog, upright; *muscles used:* hip flexors, hamstrings, quadriceps

Knee-high jog, diagonal (see figure 5.2); *muscles used:* hip flexors, hamstrings, quadriceps, core stabilizers

▶ **CUEING TIPS:** Keep the spine aligned as you lean 45 degrees to the side. Keep shoulders and hips squared, and avoid turning to the side. Pump arms from the shoulders, or scull arms down at the sides.

Knee-high jog, side-lying; *muscles used:* obliques, hip flexors, hamstrings, quadriceps

▶ **CUEING TIP:** Extend arms side to side and use only the legs.

Rock climb (see figure 5.3; hip extension); *muscle used:* gluteus maximus

▶ **CUEING TIP:** Lean forward, press heels back, reach out with arms.

Knee-high jog, faster; *muscles used:* hip flexors, hamstrings, quadriceps

▶ **CUEING TIP:** Don't lose your range of motion.

Sprint; *muscles used:* hip flexors, hamstrings, quadriceps

▶ **CUEING TIPS:** Jog faster and with more power. Pump arms from the shoulders.

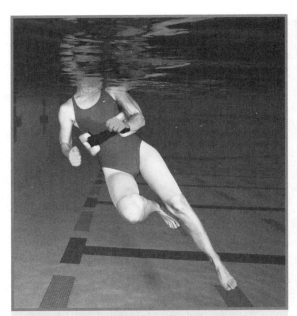

FIGURE 5.2 Knee-high jog, diagonal: Keep the spine aligned as you lean 45 degrees to the side.

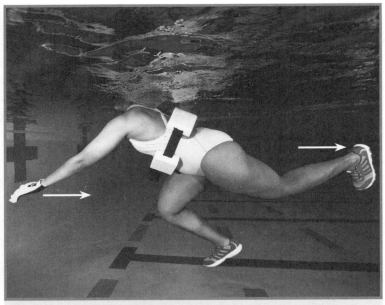

FIGURE 5.3 Rock climb: Perform a climbing motion pressing the heels back.

Knee-high jog, hands up; *muscles used:* hip flexors, hamstrings, quadriceps

▶ **CUEING TIP:** Avoid raising your hands overhead if you have high blood pressure.

Knee-high jog with elevation (see figure 5.4); *muscles used:* hip flexors, hamstrings, quadriceps

▶ **CUEING TIP:** Scull to lift the shoulders out of the water.

Steep climb (see figure 5.5); *muscles used:* hip flexors, hamstrings, quadriceps

▶ **CUEING TIPS:** Elbows are straight but not locked, press down. The motion is like climbing a ladder. Use power.

Knee-high jog, one knee only; *muscles used:* hip flexors, hamstrings, quadriceps

▶ **CUEING TIP:** Keep one leg stationary; lift the other knee up and down.

Knee-high jog, doubles; *muscles used:* hip flexors, hamstrings, quadriceps

▶ **CUEING TIP:** Lift each knee 2×.

Jump rope; *muscles used:* hip flexors, hamstrings, quadriceps, core stabilizers

▶ **CUEING TIP:** Add arm circles as if turning the rope.

Crossover knees (see figure 5.6); *muscles used:* hip flexors, hamstrings, quadriceps, obliques

▶ **CUEING TIP:** Hips twist, but trunk stays squared.

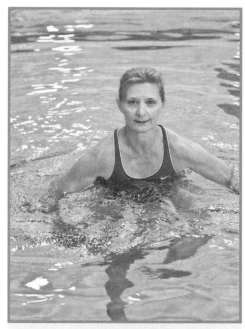

FIGURE 5.4 **Knee-high jog with elevation: Scull to lift the shoulders out of the water.**

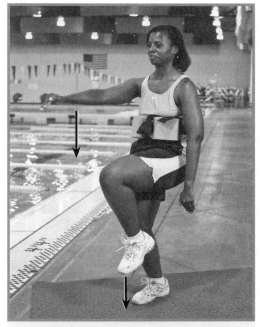

FIGURE 5.5 **Steep climb: Jog using power and power press down the arms.**

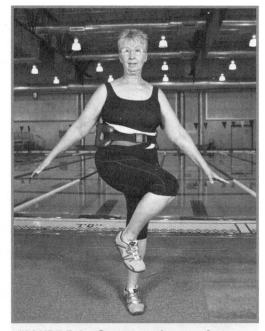

FIGURE 5.6 **Crossover knees: Jog with the knee crossing the midline of the body.**

Knee-high jog; travel forward, backward, or sideways

▶ **CUEING TIP:** Use any travel-assisting upper-body move or knee-high jog diagonally.

Sprint, travel forward

Knee-high jog, side-lying, travel sideways

Jump rope, travel forward or backward; *muscles used:* core stabilizers

▶ **CUEING TIP:** Use jump rope arms.

Knee-high jog with quick change of direction; *muscles used:* core stabilizers

Knee-high jog, travel in a circle

Knee-high jog, travel in a square

Knee-high jog, travel in a zigzag

Knee-high jog, travel in a scatter pattern

Straddle jog (see figure 5.7; hip abduction and knee flexion); *muscles used:* gluteus medius, hip adductors, hamstrings, quadriceps

▶ **CUEING TIP:** Hips are open, but feet are close together and under the body.

Straddle jog, upright; *muscles used:* gluteus medius, hip adductors, hamstrings, quadriceps

Straddle jog, diagonal; *muscles used:* gluteus medius, hip adductors, hamstrings, quadriceps, core stabilizers

▶ **CUEING TIPS:** Keep the spine aligned as you lean 45 degrees to the side. Keep shoulders and hips squared, and avoid turning to the side. Scull arms down at the sides.

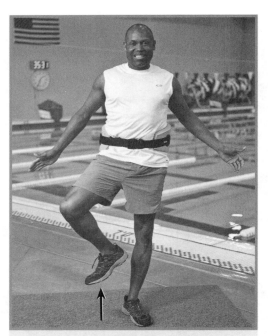

FIGURE 5.7 Straddle jog: Jog with the hips abducted and the feet under the body; push the heels down to the floor.

Seated leg press (see figure 5.8; hip and knee extension); *muscles used:* quadriceps, gluteus maximus

▶ **CUEING TIPS:** Sit in a capital letter L position. Push heels forward; point toes slightly out.

Straddle jog, faster; *muscles used:* gluteus medius, hip adductors, hamstrings, quadriceps

▶ **CUEING TIP:** Don't lose your range of motion.

Straddle jog, hands up; *muscles used:* gluteus medius, hip adductors, hamstrings, quadriceps

▶ **CUEING TIP:** Avoid raising your hands overhead if you have high blood pressure.

Straddle jog with elevation; *muscles used:* gluteus medius, hip adductors, hamstrings, quadriceps

▶ **CUEING TIP:** Scull to lift the shoulders out of the water.

Diamonds (see figure 5.9); *muscles used:* gluteus medius, hip adductors, hamstrings, quadriceps, core stabilizers

▶ **CUEING TIP:** Keep the heels together.

Diamonds, upright; *muscles used:* gluteus medius, hip adductors, hamstrings, quadriceps, core stabilizers

▶ **CUEING TIP:** Feet are under the body.

Diamonds, seated; *muscles used:* tensor fasciae latae, hip adductors, hamstrings, quadriceps, core stabilizers

▶ **CUEING TIP:** Sit in a capital letter L position.

Diamonds, upright and seated, alternate; *muscles used:* gluteus medius, tensor fasciae latae, hip adductors, hamstrings, quadriceps, core stabilizers

Straddle jog; travel forward, backward, or sideways

▶ **CUEING TIP:** Use any travel-assisting upper-body move or straddle jog diagonally.

Seated leg press, travel forward or backward

▶ **CUEING TIP:** Use scull or unison paddle pull.

Run tires (see figure 5.10; hip abduction and knee flexion); *muscles used:* gluteus medius, hip adductors, hamstrings, quadriceps

▶ **CUEING TIPS:** Hips are open and feet are wide apart; push the heels down toward the floor, as if running through tires at football practice.

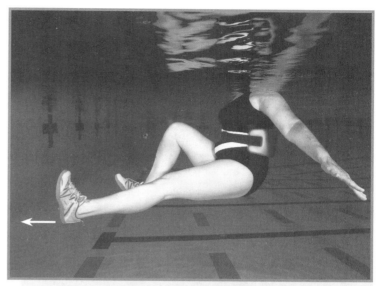

FIGURE 5.8 Seated leg press: Push the heels forward one foot at a time.

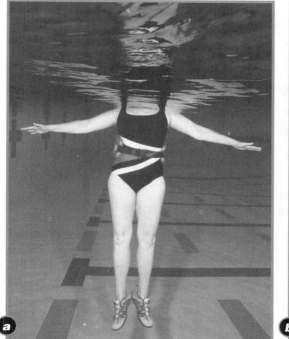 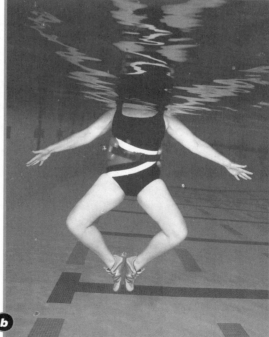

FIGURE 5.9 Diamonds: (a) Begin in the neutral position with the shoulders abducted; (b) pull the legs up in a diamond position and bring the arms down.

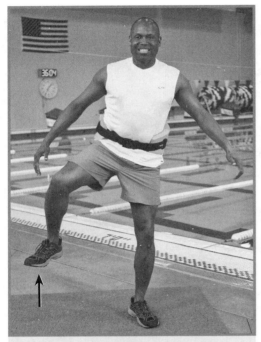

FIGURE 5.10 **Run tires: Jog with the hips abducted and the feet wide.**

Run tires, faster; *muscles used:* gluteus medius, hip adductors, hamstrings, quadriceps

▶ **CUEING TIP:** Don't lose your range of motion.

Run tires, hands up; *muscles used:* gluteus medius, hip adductors, hamstrings, quadriceps

▶ **CUEING TIP:** Avoid raising your hands overhead if you have high blood pressure.

Run tires with elevation; *muscles used:* gluteus medius, hip adductors, hamstrings, quadriceps

▶ **CUEING TIP:** Scull to lift the shoulders out of the water.

Frog kick (see figure 5.11); *muscles used:* gluteus medius, hip adductors, hamstrings, quadriceps

▶ **CUEING TIPS:** Lift the knees wide; then straighten the legs and pull them together. Pull the arms and legs together forcefully to lift the shoulders out of the water.

In in, out out; *muscles used:* gluteus medius, hip adductors, hamstrings, quadriceps

▶ **CUEING TIP:** Jog, alternate feet in and out.

Over the barrel, travel sideways (see figure 5.12); *muscles used:* gluteus medius, hip adductors, hamstrings, quadriceps

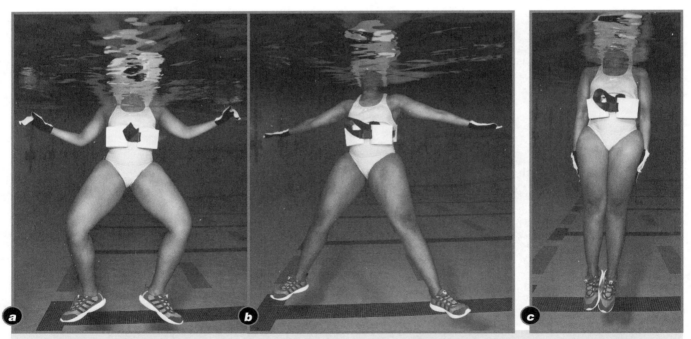

FIGURE 5.11 **Frog kick:** *(a)* **Begin by abducting the hips and flexing the knees;** *(b)* **straighten the legs;** *(c)* **pull them together.**

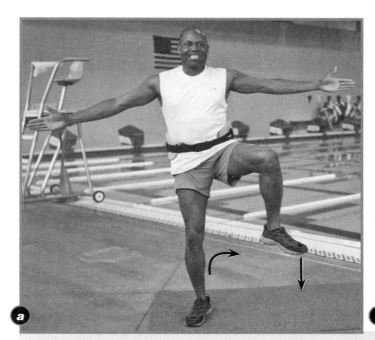 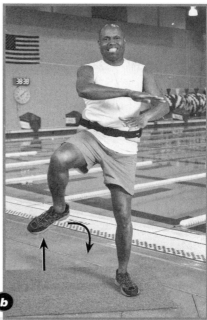

FIGURE 5.12 **Over the barrel, travel sideways:** *(a)* Travel sideways as if stepping over a barrel with one foot; *(b)* then step over it with the other foot.

▶ **CUEING TIPS:** Travel sideways as if stepping over barrels one foot at a time. Use sidestroke.

Run tires; travel forward, backward, or sideways

▶ **CUEING TIP:** Use any travel-assisting upper-body move.

Ankle touch (see figure 5.13; hip flexion and lateral rotation); *muscles used:* hip flexors, tensor fasciae latae, sartorius

▶ **CUEING TIPS:** Bring the ankle up to the hand; bring the hand down to the ankle. If you can't reach the ankle, aim for the shin or knee instead.

Ankle touch, faster; *muscles used:* hip flexors, tensor fasciae latae, sartorius

▶ **CUEING TIP:** Don't lose your range of motion.

Ankle touch, feet close together or wide apart; *muscles used:* hip flexors, tensor fasciae latae, sartorius

Ankle touch, one ankle only; *muscles used:* hip flexors, tensor fasciae latae, sartorius

Ankle touch, doubles; *muscles used:* hip flexors, tensor fasciae latae, sartorius, core stabilizers

▶ **CUEING TIP:** Touch each ankle 2×.

Ankle touch, travel forward

▶ **CUEING TIP:** Emphasize the downward movement of both arms and legs.

Ankle touch, travel backward

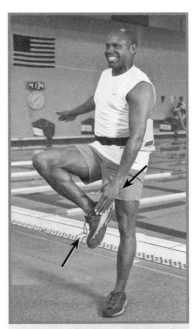

FIGURE 5.13 **Ankle touch: Touch the ankle with the opposite hand.**

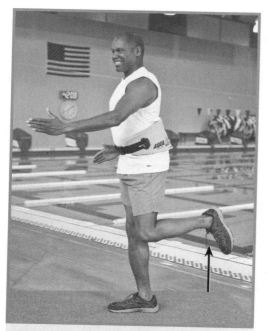

FIGURE 5.14 **Heel jog: Jog with a heel lift in back.**

▶ **CUEING TIP:** Emphasize the upward movement of both arms and legs.

Heel jog (see figure 5.14; knee flexion); *muscles used:* hamstrings, quadriceps

▶ **CUEING TIP:** Keep knees under hips and curl the hamstrings.

Heel jog, upright; *muscles used:* hamstrings, quadriceps

Heel jog, diagonal; *muscles used:* hamstrings, quadriceps, core stabilizers

▶ **CUEING TIPS:** Keep the spine aligned as you lean 45 degrees to the side. Keep shoulders and hips squared, and avoid turning to the side. Scull arms down at the sides.

Heel jog, faster; *muscles used:* hamstrings, quadriceps

▶ **CUEING TIP:** Don't lose your range of motion.

Heel jog, hands up; *muscles used:* hamstrings, quadriceps

▶ **CUEING TIP:** Avoid raising your hands overhead if you have high blood pressure.

Heel jog with elevation; *muscles used:* hamstrings, quadriceps

▶ **CUEING TIP:** Scull to lift the shoulders out of the water.

Breaststroke kick (see figure 5.15); *muscles used:* hamstrings, quadriceps, gluteus medius, hip adductors

▶ **CUEING TIPS:** Lift the heels in back; then straighten the legs with the feet apart and pull them together. Pull the arms and legs together forcefully to lift the shoulders out of the water.

Heel jog, feet close together or wide apart; *muscles used:* hamstrings, quadriceps

Heel jog, one heel only; *muscles used:* hamstrings, quadriceps

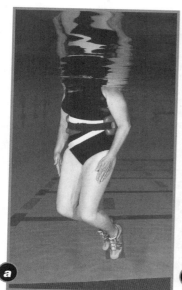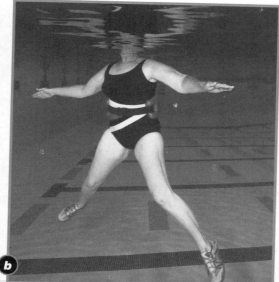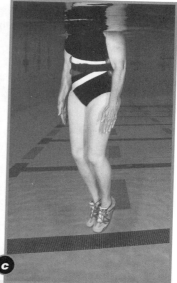

FIGURE 5.15 **Breaststroke kick:** *(a)* Begin by lifting the heels; *(b)* straighten the legs with the feet apart; *(c)* pull them together.

▶ **CUEING TIP:** Keep one leg stationary; lift the other heel up and down in back.

Heel jog, doubles; *muscles used:* hamstrings, quadriceps

▶ **CUEING TIP:** Lift each heel 2×.

Heel jog; travel forward, backward, or sideways

▶ **CUEING TIP:** Use any travel-assisting upper-body move or heel jog diagonally.

Hopscotch (see figure 5.16; knee flexion); *muscles used:* hamstrings, quadriceps

▶ **CUEING TIPS:** Touch the heel in back with the opposite hand. If you can't touch the heel, just aim for it.

Hopscotch, faster; *muscles used:* hamstrings, quadriceps

▶ **CUEING TIP:** Don't lose your range of motion.

Hopscotch, feet close together or wide apart; *muscles used:* hamstrings, quadriceps

Hopscotch, one heel only; *muscles used:* hamstrings, quadriceps

Hopscotch, doubles; *muscles used:* hamstrings, quadriceps

▶ **CUEING TIP:** Touch each heel 2×.

Hopscotch, travel forward

▶ **CUEING TIP:** Emphasize the upward movement of the legs.

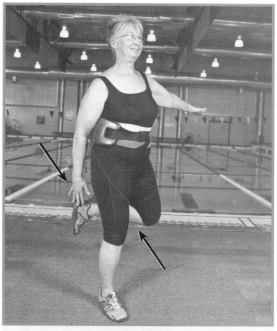

FIGURE 5.16 **Hopscotch: Touch the heel in back with the opposite hand.**

BICYCLE

Bicycle (see figure 5.17; hip and knee flexion and extension); *muscles used:* hip flexors, hamstrings, quadriceps

▶ **CUEING TIP:** Keep the feet under the body as if riding a unicycle.

Bicycle, upright; *muscles used:* hip flexors, hamstrings, quadriceps

Bicycle, diagonal; *muscles used:* hip flexors, hamstrings, quadriceps, core stabilizers

▶ **CUEING TIPS:** Keep the spine aligned as you lean 45 degrees to the side. Keep shoulders and hips squared, and avoid turning to the side. Scull arms down at the sides.

Bicycle, side-lying; *muscles used:* obliques, hip flexors, hamstrings, quadriceps

▶ **CUEING TIP:** Extend arms side to side and use only the legs.

Bicycle, side-lying in a circle; *muscles used:* obliques, hip flexors, hamstrings, quadriceps

▶ **CUEING TIPS:** Pedal the feet in big circles. Extend arms side to side and use only the legs.

Seated bicycle; *muscles used:* hip flexors, hamstrings, quadriceps

▶ **CUEING TIP:** As if on a recumbent bicycle.

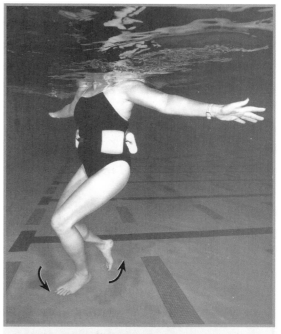

FIGURE 5.17 **Bicycle: Pedal the feet in a circular motion.**

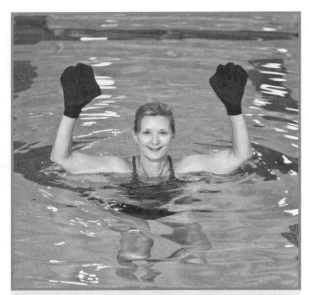

FIGURE 5.18 Bicycle, hands up: Hold the hands up to make the legs work harder.

Bicycle, faster; *muscles used:* hip flexors, hamstrings, quadriceps

▶ **CUEING TIP:** Don't lose your range of motion.

Bicycle, hands up (see figure 5.18); *muscles used:* hip flexors, hamstrings, quadriceps

▶ **CUEING TIP:** Avoid raising your hands overhead if you have high blood pressure.

Bicycle with elevation; *muscles used:* hip flexors, hamstrings, quadriceps

▶ **CUEING TIP:** Scull to lift the shoulders out of the water.

Bicycle, large or small circles; *muscles used:* hip flexors, hamstrings, quadriceps

Bicycle, climb a hill; *muscles used:* hip flexors, hamstrings, quadriceps

▶ **CUEING TIPS:** Put your bicycle in first gear and climb a hill. Use power.

Bicycle, one leg only; *muscles used:* hip flexors, hamstrings, quadriceps, core stabilizers

▶ **CUEING TIP:** Keep one leg stationary; bicycle with the other leg.

Bicycle, tandem; *muscles used:* hip flexors, hamstrings, quadriceps, core stabilizers

▶ **CUEING TIP:** Bicycle with legs in unison.

Bicycle, reverse; *muscles used:* hip flexors, hamstrings, quadriceps

▶ **CUEING TIP:** Pedal in reverse.

Bicycle, travel forward

▶ **CUEING TIP:** Travel without using the arms or use any travel-assisting upper-body move.

Bicycle, travel backward

▶ **CUEING TIP:** Pedal in reverse or use any backward travel-assisting upper-body move.

Bicycle, travel sideways

▶ **CUEING TIP:** Use any sideways travel-assisting upper-body move or bicycle diagonally.

Bicycle, side-lying, travel sideways

KICK

Flutter kick (see figure 5.19; hip flexion); *muscles used:* hip flexors, gluteus maximus

▶ **CUEING TIPS:** Flutter kick from the hips, not the knees. Floppy feet. Maintain upright posture with shoulders, hips, and feet in alignment.

Flutter kick, upright; *muscles used:* hip flexors, gluteus maximus

Flutter kick, diagonal; *muscles used:* hip flexors, gluteus maximus, core stabilizers

▶ **CUEING TIPS:** Keep the spine aligned as you lean 45 degrees to the side. Keep shoulders and hips squared, and avoid turning to the side. Scull arms down at the sides.

Flutter kick, side-lying; *muscles used:* obliques, hip flexors, gluteus maximus

▶ **CUEING TIP:** Extend arms side to side and use only the legs.

Seated flutter kick; *muscles used:* hip flexors, gluteus maximus

▶ **CUEING TIP:** Sit in a capital letter L position.

Flutter kick, faster; *muscles used:* hip flexors, gluteus maximus

Flutter kick, hands up; *muscles used:* hip flexors, gluteus maximus

▶ **CUEING TIP:** Avoid raising your hands overhead if you have high blood pressure.

Flutter kick with elevation; *muscles used:* hip flexors, gluteus maximus

▶ **CUEING TIP:** Scull to lift the shoulders out of the water.

Flutter kick, feet pointed or flexed; *muscles used:* hip flexors, gluteus maximus, gastrocnemius, tibilias anterior

Flutter kick, one leg only; *muscles used:* hip flexors, gluteus maximus, core stabilizers

▶ **CUEING TIP:** Keep one leg stationary; flutter kick with the other leg.

Flutter kick up to L position and down to upright (see figure 5.20); *muscles used:* hip flexors, gluteus maximus, core stabilizers

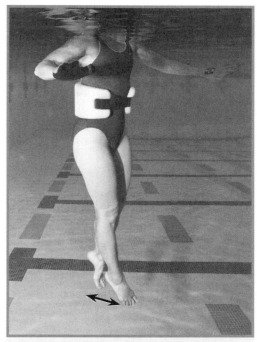

FIGURE 5.19 **Flutter kick: Flutter kick from the hips.**

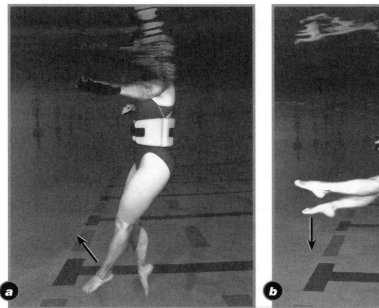 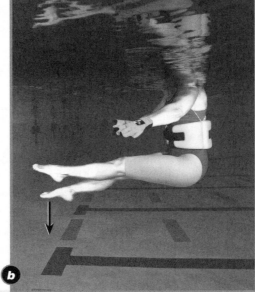

FIGURE 5.20 **Flutter kick up to L position and down to upright:** *(a)* **Begin the flutter kick in neutral posture;** *(b)* **walk the flutter kick up to the L position.**

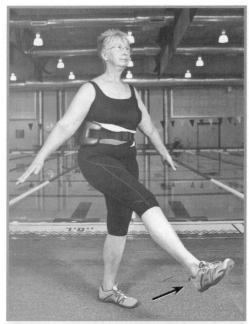

FIGURE 5.21 Kick forward: Kick forward with soft knees.

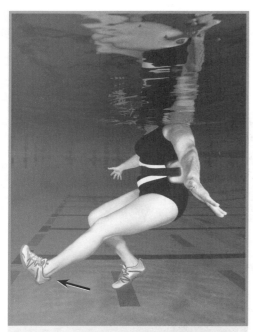

FIGURE 5.22 Seated kick: Kick from the knees in a seated position.

Flutter kick, travel forward, backward or sideways

▶ **CUEING TIP:** Use any travel-assisting upper-body move or flutter kick diagonally.

Flutter kick, side-lying, travel sideways

Kick forward (see figure 5.21; hip flexion and knee extension); *muscles used:* hip flexors, quadriceps, hamstrings

▶ **CUEING TIPS:** Keep knees soft. Return the legs under the body after each kick.

Kick forward, upright; *muscles used:* hip flexors, quadriceps, hamstrings

Seated kick (see figure 5.22); *muscles used:* quadriceps, hamstrings

▶ **CUEING TIPS:** Sit in a dining room chair position. Participants with knee problems may wish to substitute a seated leg press for the seated kick.

Mermaid–unison kick; *muscles used:* quadriceps, hamstrings, core stabilizers

▶ **CUEING TIP:** Like pumping a swing.

Kick forward, faster; *muscles used:* hip flexors, quadriceps, hamstrings

▶ **CUEING TIP:** Don't lose your range of motion.

High kick; *muscles used:* hip flexors, gluteus maximus

▶ **CUEING TIP:** Maintain your upright posture while kicking forward using your full range of motion.

High kick 7×, tuck and turn; *muscles used:* hip flexors, gluteus maximus, core stabilizers

▶ **CUEING TIP:** 7 high kicks, then tuck and half turn.

One leg kicks forward; *muscles used:* hip flexors, gluteus maximus, core stabilizers

▶ **CUEING TIP:** Keep one leg stationary; lift the other leg up and down in front.

Kick forward, doubles; *muscles used:* hip flexors, gluteus maximus, core stabilizers

▶ **CUEING TIP:** Lift each leg 2×.

Crossover kick (see figure 5.23); *muscles used:* hip flexors, quadriceps, hamstrings, obliques

▶ **CUEING TIP:** Kick across the body.

Kick to the corners; *muscles used:* gluteus medius, quadriceps, hamstrings

Kick forward; travel forward, backward, or sideways

▶ **CUEING TIP:** Use any travel-assisting upper-body move.

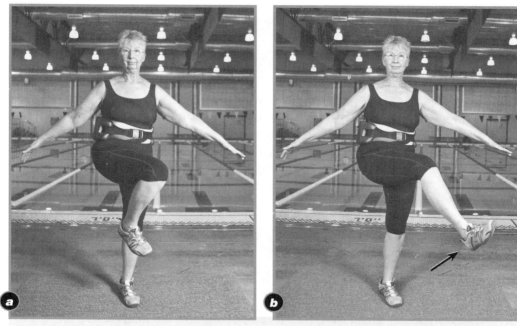

FIGURE 5.23 **Crossover kick:** *(a)* **Lift the knee;** *(b)* **kick with the leg crossing the midline of the body.**

Seated kick, travel forward

▶ **CUEING TIP:** Flex the feet and emphasize the knee flexion.

Seated kick, travel backward

▶ **CUEING TIP:** Point the toes and emphasize the knee extension.

High kick, travel forward

▶ **CUEING TIP:** Emphasize the downward movement of both arms and legs.

High kick, travel backward

▶ **CUEING TIP:** Emphasize the upward movement of both arms and legs.

Cossack kick (see figure 5.24; hip abduction and knee flexion and extension); *muscles used:* gluteus medius, quadriceps, hamstrings

▶ **CUEING TIP:** Bring legs into a diamond position under the body and kick to the sides.

Cossack kick, upright; *muscles used:* gluteus medius, quadriceps, hamstrings

Cossack kick, diagonal; *muscles used:* gluteus medius, quadriceps, hamstrings, core stabilizers

▶ **CUEING TIPS:** Keep the spine aligned as you lean 45 degrees to the side. Keep shoulders and hips squared, and avoid turning to the side. Scull arms down at the sides.

Seated Cossack kick; *muscles used:* gluteus medius, quadriceps, hamstrings

▶ **CUEING TIP:** Sit with the legs in a diamond position and kick to the sides.

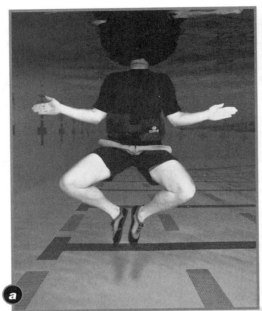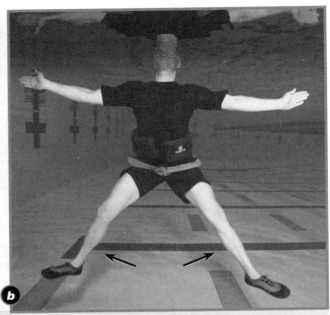

FIGURE 5.24 Cossack kick: *(a)* Begin with the hips abducted and the heels together; *(b)* kick from the knees out to the sides.

Cossack kick, faster; *muscles used:* gluteus medius, quadriceps, hamstrings

▶ **CUEING TIP:** Don't lose your range of motion.

Cossack kick with alternating legs; *muscles used:* gluteus medius, quadriceps, hamstrings

One leg kicks side; *muscles used:* gluteus medius, hip adductors, core stabilizers

Cossack kick, travel sideways

▶ **CUEING TIP:** Use sidestroke.

Skate kick (see figure 5.25; hip extension); *muscle used:* gluteus maximus

▶ **CUEING TIPS:** Kick backward with the leg straight. Tighten the glutes.

Skate kick, faster; *muscle used:* gluteus maximus

▶ **CUEING TIP:** Don't lose your range of motion.

Skate kick, higher; *muscle used:* gluteus maximus

Skate kick with power; *muscle used:* gluteus maximus

One leg kicks back; *muscles used:* gluteus maximus, core stabilizers

▶ **CUEING TIP:** Keep one leg stationary; lift the other leg up and down in back.

Skate kick, travel forward

▶ **CUEING TIP:** Use breaststroke or hands behind back.

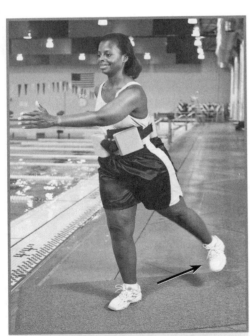

FIGURE 5.25 Skate kick: Kick backward with the leg straight.

Skate kick, travel backward

▶ **CUEING TIP:** Use reverse breaststroke.

CROSS-COUNTRY SKI

Cross-country ski (see figure 5.26; hip flexion and extension); *muscles used:* gluteus maximus, hip flexors

▶ **CUEING TIPS:** Balance the body by working the arms and legs in opposition. Swing legs and arms forward and backward evenly. Look over your shoulder to make sure the legs are going to the back.

Cross-country ski, upright; *muscles used:* gluteus maximus, hip flexors

Cross-country ski, knees bent 90 degrees (see figure 5.27); *muscles used:* gluteus maximus, hip flexors, hamstrings

▶ **CUEING TIPS:** Knees bent makes a short lever cross-country ski, which is less intense. Scull or use an arm swing.

Cross-country ski, diagonal; *muscles used:* gluteus maximus, hip flexors, core stabilizers

▶ **CUEING TIPS:** Keep the spine aligned as you lean 45 degrees to the side. Keep shoulders and hips squared, and avoid turning to the side. Arms swing forward and back.

Cross-country ski, side-lying; *muscles used:* obliques, gluteus maximus, hip flexors

▶ **CUEING TIP:** Extend arms side to side and use only the legs.

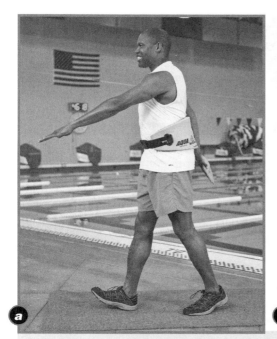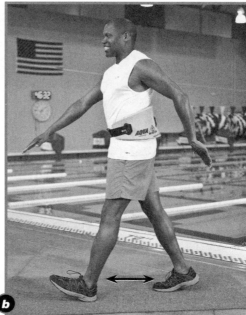

FIGURE 5.26 Cross-country ski: *(a)* **Begin with the right leg and the left arm forward;** *(b)* **switch to the left leg and right arm forward.**

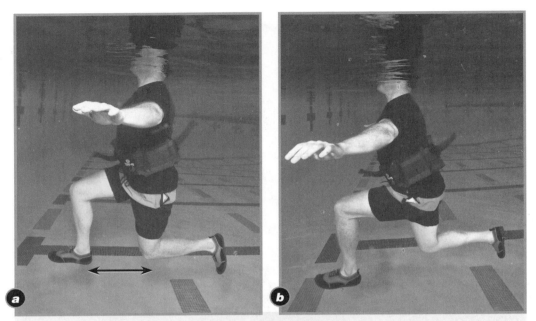

FIGURE 5.27 **Cross-country ski, knees bent 90 degrees:** *(a)* **Begin with the right leg forward and both knees bent;** *(b)* **switch to the left leg forward.**

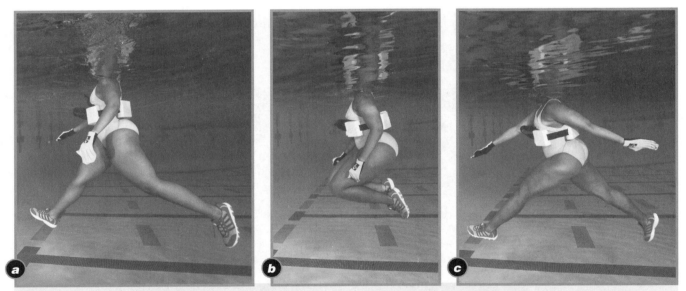

FIGURE 5.28 **Tuck ski:** *(a)* **Begin with the right leg and the left arm forward;** *(b)* **tuck the feet under the body;** *(c)* **complete the move with the left leg and the right arm forward.**

Tuck ski (see figure 5.28); *muscles used:* gluteus maximus, hip flexors, core stabilizers

Tuck ski together (see figure 5.29); *muscles used:* gluteus maximus, hip flexors, core stabilizers

▶ **CUEING TIP:** Tuck, ski, and pull the legs together forcefully to lift the shoulders out of the water.

Cross-country ski, faster; *muscles used:* gluteus maximus, hip flexors

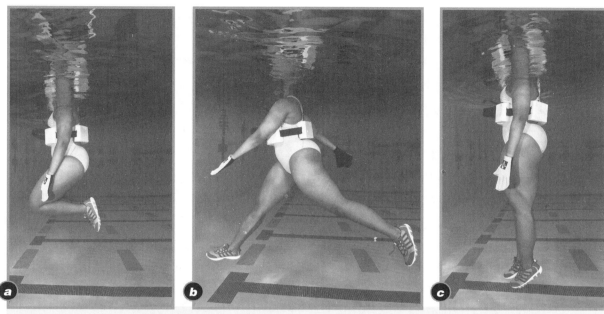

FIGURE 5.29 **Tuck ski together:** *(a)* **Begin by tucking the feet under the body;** *(b)* **go into a cross-country ski;** *(c)* **pull the legs together forcefully.**

▷ **CUEING TIP:** Don't lose your range of motion.

Mini ski; *muscles used:* gluteus maximus, hip flexors

▷ **CUEING TIP:** Short and tight and fast.

Cross-country ski, full range of motion; *muscles used:* gluteus maximus, hip flexors

Cross-country ski with elevation; *muscles used:* gluteus maximus, hip flexors

▷ **CUEING TIP:** Pull the arms and legs together forcefully to lift the shoulders out of the water.

Cross-country ski with power; *muscles used:* gluteus maximus, hip flexors

Cross-country ski, corner to corner (see figure 5.30); *muscles used:* gluteus maximus, hip flexors, obliques

▷ **CUEING TIPS:** Reach the arm across the chest. Reach across R, stop in the center, and reach across L. Increase intensity by eliminating the stop in the center.

Tuck ski, corner to corner; *muscles used:* gluteus maximus, hip flexors, core stabilizers

▷ **CUEING TIP:** Reach across R, tuck the feet under the body, and reach across L.

Cross-country ski with quarter turn; *muscles used:* gluteus maximus, hip flexors

▷ **CUEING TIP:** Ski 2-8×; then turn.

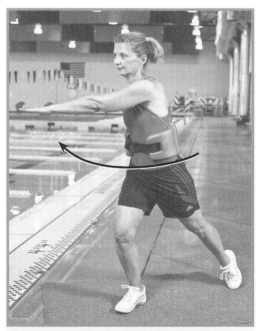

FIGURE 5.30 **Cross-country ski, corner to corner: Reach the left arm across the midline of the body as the left leg extends toward the opposite corner.**

Cross-country ski 3 1/2×, half turn; *muscles used:* gluteus maximus, hip flexors

▶ **CUEING TIP:** Ski R, L, R, L, R, L, R, and turn.

Cross-country ski, travel forward

▶ **CUEING TIP:** Scoop the arms back with power and slice forward.

Cross-country ski, travel backward

▶ **CUEING TIP:** Scoop the arms forward with power and slice backward.

Cross-country ski, travel sideways

▶ **CUEING TIP:** Use unison sidestroke or cross-country ski diagonally.

Cross-country ski, side-lying; tuck ski together, side-lying, travel sideways

JUMPING JACKS

Jumping jacks (see figure 5.31; hip abduction and adduction); *muscles used:* gluteus medius, hip adductors

▶ **CUEING TIP:** Arms opposite legs or extended to sides to prevent bobbing.

Jumping jacks, upright: *muscles used:* gluteus medius, hip adductors

Seated jacks (horizontal hip abduction and adduction); *muscles used:* tensor fasciae latae, hip adductors

▶ **CUEING TIP:** Sit in a capital letter L position.

Seated jacks with toes in or out; *muscles used:* gluteus medius, hip adductors

Seated jacks, 45 degrees; *muscles used:* gluteus medius, hip adductors, core stabilizers

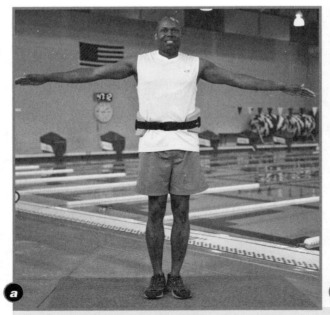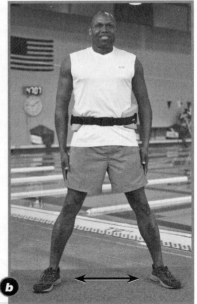

FIGURE 5.31 **Jumping jacks:** *(a)* **Begin with the shoulders abducted and the feet together;** *(b)* **bring the feet apart as the arms come down.**

▶ **CUEING TIP:** Legs are halfway between upright and seated.

Jumping jacks, side-lying (see figure 5.32); *muscles used:* obliques, gluteus medius, hip adductors

▶ **CUEING TIP:** Extend arms side to side and use only the legs.

Jacks tuck (see figure 5.33); *muscles used:* gluteus medius, core stabilizers

Jumping jacks, faster; *muscles used:* gluteus medius, hip adductors

▶ **CUEING TIP:** Don't lose your range of motion.

Mini jacks; *muscles used:* gluteus medius, hip adductors

▶ **CUEING TIP:** Short and tight and fast.

Mini cross; *muscles used:* gluteus medius, hip adductors

▶ **CUEING TIP:** Cross the legs in a short motion.

Triple crossover; *muscles used:* gluteus medius, hip adductors

▶ **CUEING TIP:** Mini cross 3×, jack 1×.

Jacks cross (see figure 5.34); *muscles used:* gluteus medius, hip adductors

Jacks cross, full range of motion; *muscles used:* gluteus medius, hip adductors

Jumping jacks with power; *muscles used:* gluteus medius, hip adductors

Jumping jacks with quarter turn; *muscles used:* gluteus medius, hip adductors

▶ **CUEING TIP:** Jumping jacks 2–8×; then turn.

Jacks cross, 3 1/2×, half turn; *muscles used:* gluteus medius, hip adductors

▶ **CUEING TIP:** Cross, out, cross, out, cross, out, cross, and turn.

Jumping jacks, travel forward

▶ **CUEING TIP:** Clap hands, push arms apart and slice in.

Jumping jacks, travel backward

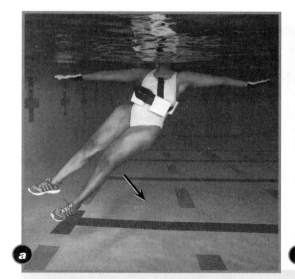 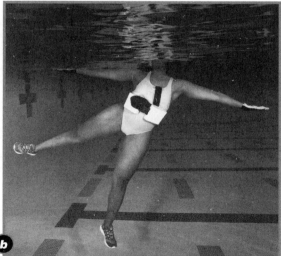

FIGURE 5.32 **Jumping jacks, side-lying:** *(a)* **Begin in the side-lying position with the legs together;** *(b)* **abduct the hips.**

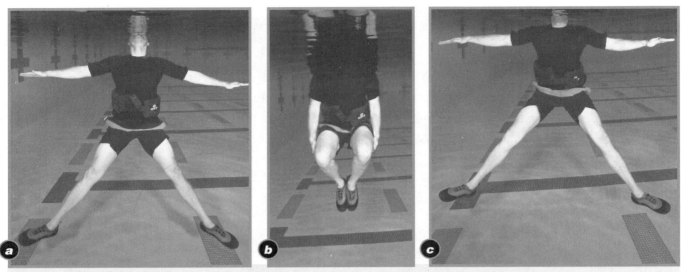

FIGURE 5.33 **Jacks tuck:** *(a)* **Begin with the shoulders abducted and the feet apart;** *(b)* **bring the arms down and tuck the feet under the body;** *(c)* **return to the starting position.**

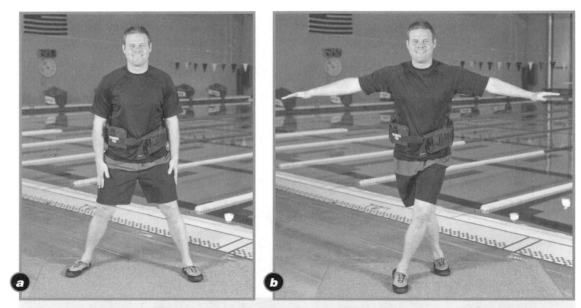

FIGURE 5.34 **Jacks cross:** *(a)* **Begin with the feet apart and the arms down;** *(b)* **abduct the shoulders and cross the legs.**

▶ **CUEING TIP:** Clap hands, pull arms together and slice out.

Jumping jacks, travel sideways

▶ **CUEING TIPS:** Arms and legs work together instead of opposite. Pull one arm and leg to center with power.

Seated jacks, travel forward or backward

▶ **CUEING TIP:** Clap hands.

TRAVEL ASSISTING UPPER-BODY MOVES

For other upper-body moves, see the shallow-water exercises in chapter 2.

Scull arms down, travel forward (see figure 5.35); *muscles used:* pronators, biceps

Scull in front, travel backward (see figure 5.36); *muscles used:* pronators, biceps

▶ **CUEING TIP:** Sweep hands out with thumbs angled down, sweep hands in with thumbs angled up, keep fingers up.

Crawl stroke, travel forward; *muscles used:* trapezius, rhomboids

▶ **CUEING TIP:** Reach and pull.

Push forward, travel backward; *muscle used:* triceps

▶ **CUEING TIP:** Push forward with the palms, pull the hands back in a slice; alternate hands.

Standing row, travel forward (see figure 5.37); *muscles used:* trapezius, rhomboids

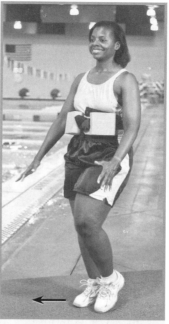

FIGURE 5.35 **Scull arms down, travel forward: Make figure eights, arms down at the sides.**

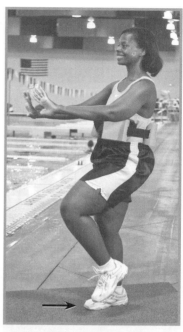

FIGURE 5.36 **Scull in front, travel backward: Keep fingers up.**

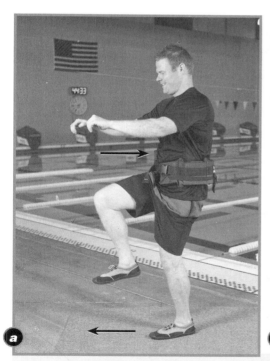

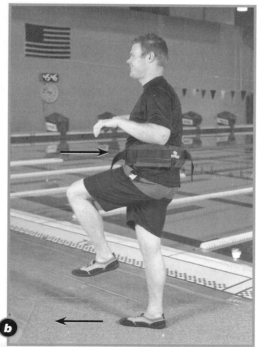

FIGURE 5.37 **Standing row, travel forward: *(a)* Begin by reaching the arms forward with hands cupped; *(b)* pull the elbows back.**

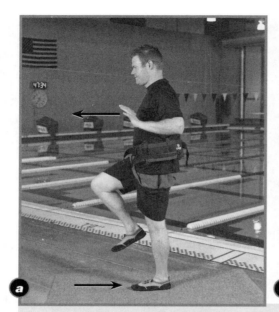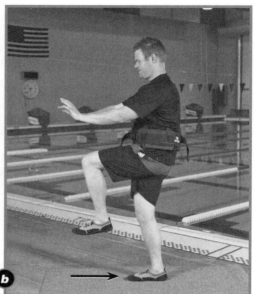

FIGURE 5.38 Unison push forward, travel backward: *(a)* Begin with the hands in front of the chest with fingers up; *(b)* push both hands forward.

Unison push forward, travel backward (see figure 5.38); *muscle used:* triceps

▶ **CUEING TIP:** Push forward with the palms, pull the hands back in a slice.

Breaststroke, travel forward; *muscles used:* pectorals, deltoids, trapezius, rhomboids

▶ **CUEING TIP:** Do breaststroke with thumbs up to protect the shoulders.

Reverse breaststroke, travel backward; *muscles used:* pectorals, trapezius, rhomboids

Clap hands, travel forward; *muscles used:* deltoids, pectorals

▶ **CUEING TIP:** Push arms apart and slice in.

Clap hands, travel backward; *muscles used:* pectorals, deltoids

▶ **CUEING TIP:** Pull arms together and slice out.

Unison arm swing, travel forward; *muscles used:* latissimus dorsi, deltoids

▶ **CUEING TIP:** Scoop backward and slice forward.

Unison arm swing, travel backward; *muscles used:* deltoids, latissimus dorsi

▶ **CUEING TIP:** Scoop forward and slice backward.

Double-arm press-down, travel forward (see figure 5.39); *muscle used:* latissimus dorsi, trapezius, triceps

▶ **CUEING TIP:** Press down, slide the hands up, reach forward, and press down again.

Double-arm lift, travel backward (see figure 5.40); *muscles used:* deltoids, trapezius, triceps

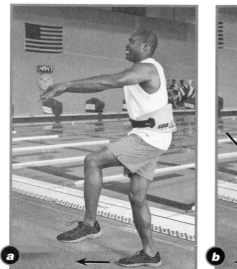
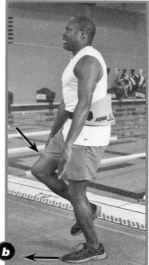
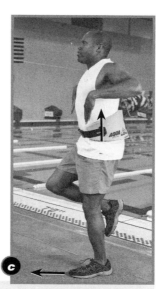

FIGURE 5.39 Double-arm press-down, travel forward: *(a)* Begin with the shoulders flexed; *(b)* press the arms down; *(c)* slide the hands up.

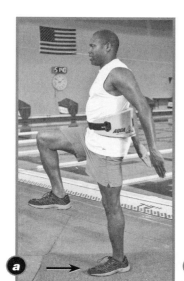
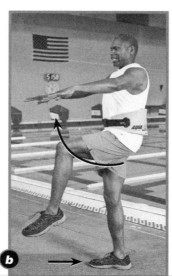
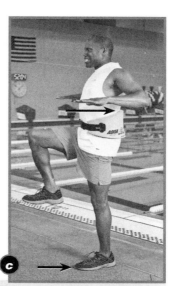

FIGURE 5.40 Double-arm lift, travel backward: *(a)* Begin with the arms down; *(b)* lift the arms in front; *(c)* pull the elbows in.

▶ **CUEING TIP:** Lift, pull the elbows in, slide the hands down, and lift again.

Forearm press out, travel forward; *muscle used:* rotator cuff

▶ **CUEING TIP:** Press out with the backs of the hands and slice in; keep the elbows glued to the waist.

Forearm press in, travel backward; *muscle used:* rotator cuff

▶ **CUEING TIP:** Press the palms in and slice out; keep the elbows glued to the waist.

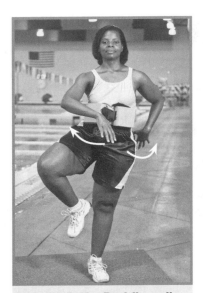

FIGURE 5.41 **Paddle pull, travel forward: Pull water from bellybutton to back with alternating arms.**

Paddle pull, travel forward (see figure 5.41); *muscles used:* trapezius, rhomboids, obliques

▶ **CUEING TIP:** Pull water from bellybutton to back with arms in unison or alternate arms.

Paddle pull, travel backward; *muscles used:* pectorals, obliques

▶ **CUEING TIP:** Pull water from back to bellybutton with arms in unison or alternate arms.

Jump rope arms, travel forward or backward; *muscles used:* biceps, triceps

Sidestroke, travel sideways; *muscles used:* deltoids, pectorals

▶ **CUEING TIPS:** Reach alternating arms to one side and pull past the midline. Keep abdominals tight to avoid leaning.

Unison sidestroke, travel sideways (see figure 5.42); *muscles used:* deltoids, pectorals

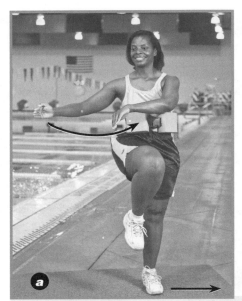 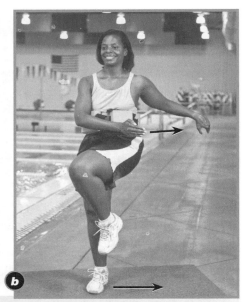

FIGURE 5.42 **Unison sidestroke, travel sideways:** *(a)* **Reach both arms to one side;** *(b)* **pull past the midline.**

▶ **CUEING TIPS:** Reach both arms to one side and pull past the midline. Keep abdominals tight to avoid leaning.

Single-arm sweep, travel sideways (see figure 5.43); *muscles used:* deltoids, pectorals

▶ **CUEING TIP:** Begin with arms out to the sides, sweep one arm toward the opposite arm.

Side arm curl, travel sideways (see figure 5.44); *muscles used:* biceps, deltoids

▶ **CUEING TIP:** Begin with arms out to the sides, bend the elbow and pull the palm toward the chest.

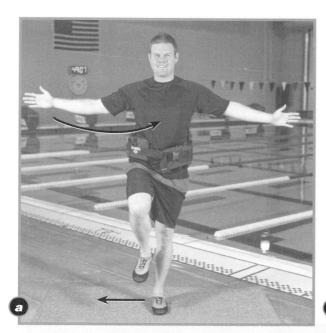
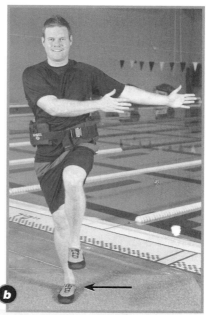

FIGURE 5.43 Single-arm sweep, travel sideways: *(a)* Begin with shoulders abducted; *(b)* sweep one arm toward the opposite arm.

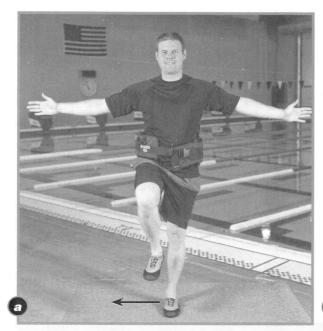
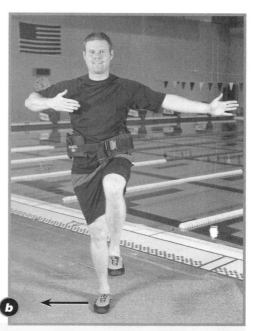

FIGURE 5.44 Side arm curl, travel sideways: *(a)* Begin with the shoulders abducted to the sides; *(b)* flex one elbow and pull the palm toward the chest.

ABDOMINALS

Trunk flexion; *muscle used:* rectus abdominis

Pelvic tilt; *muscle used:* rectus abdominis

▶ **CUEING TIP:** Upright or seated.

Crunch, V position (see figure 5.45); *muscle used:* rectus abdominis

Crunch with legs in a diamond position; *muscle used:* rectus abdominis

Eight short crunches and two long crunches; *muscle used:* rectus abdominis

V-sit; *muscle used:* rectus abdominis

▶ **CUEING TIP:** Pull chest and straight legs together.

The hundred (Pilates); *muscle used:* rectus abdominis

▶ **CUEING TIP:** Hold V and pulse hands at sides.

Hold V and scull to travel forward; *muscle used:* rectus abdominis

Rolling like a ball (Pilates); *muscle used:* rectus abdominis

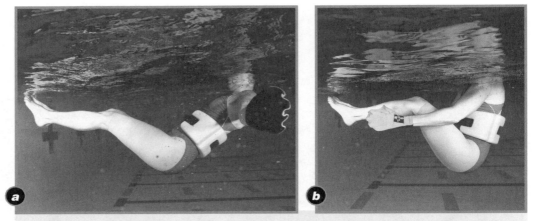

FIGURE 5.45 **Crunch, V position: *(a)* Begin in the V position; *(b)* pull the chest toward the knees.**

▶ **CUEING TIP:** Pull knees to chest and roll from reclining to seated with scull.

Abdominal pike (see figure 5.46); *muscles used:* rectus abdominis, hip flexors

▶ **CUEING TIP:** Begin in an upright position, tuck the feet under the body, and then extend the legs forward in an abdominal pike.

Abdominal pike and spine extension (see figure 5.47); *muscles used:* rectus abdominis, erector spinae

▶ **CUEING TIPS:** Begin with the legs extended forward, tuck the feet under the body, and extend legs back at a 45 degree angle. Extend legs back at a 45-degree angle to avoid hyperextending the back or neck. Keep legs together. Participants with low back pain may wish to substitute abdominal pike for abdominal pike and spine extension.

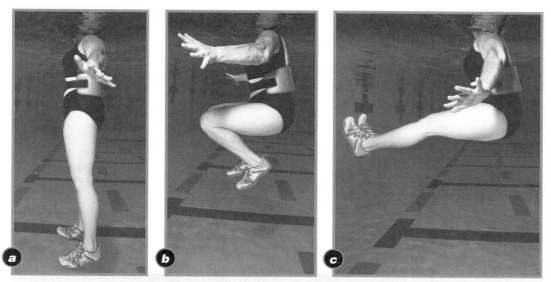

FIGURE 5.46 Abdominal pike: *(a)* Begin in neutral posture; *(b)* tuck the feet under the body; *(c)* extend the legs forward in an abdominal pike.

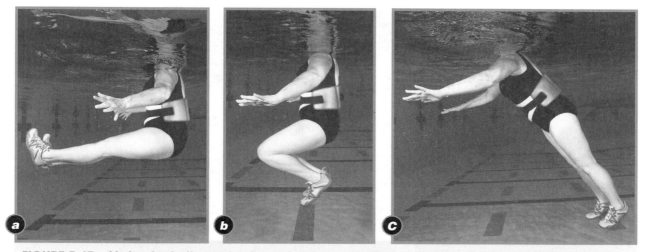

FIGURE 5.47 Abdominal pike and spine extension: *(a)* Begin in the abdominal pike position; *(b)* tuck the feet under the body; *(c)* extend the legs to the back at a 45 degree angle.

Abdominal pike and spine extension, legs wide in front and together in back; *muscles used:* rectus abdominis, erector spinae

Abdominal pike and spine extension, legs together in front and wide in back; *muscles used:* rectus abdominis, erector spinae

Abdominal pike and spine extension, legs wide in front and wide in back with tuck in center; *muscles used:* rectus abdominis, erector spinae

Abdominal pike and spine extension with legs in a diamond position; *muscles used:* rectus abdominis, erector spinae

Hip flexion; *muscles used:* hip flexors, abdominals stabilize

Hip curl; *muscles used:* hip flexors, abdominals stabilize

▶ **CUEING TIP:** Pull knees to chest.

Hip curl from a kneeling position; *muscles used:* hip flexors, abdominals stabilize

Hip curl, L position (see figure 5.48); *muscles used:* hip flexors, abdominals stabilize

Hip curl, V position; *muscles used:* hip flexors, abdominals stabilize

Hip curl with unison or alternating knees; *muscles used:* hip flexors, abdominals stabilize

Hip curl with one foot on top of the other; *muscles used:* hip flexors, abdominals stabilize

Hip curl with legs in a diamond position; *muscles used:* tensor fasciae latae, abdominals stabilize

Single-leg stretch (Pilates; see figure 5.49); *muscles used:* hip flexors, abdominals stabilize

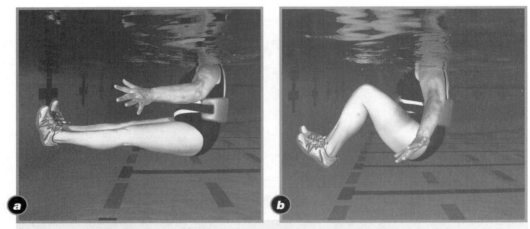

FIGURE 5.48 **Hip curl, L position: *(a)* Begin in the L position; *(b)* pull knees to chest.**

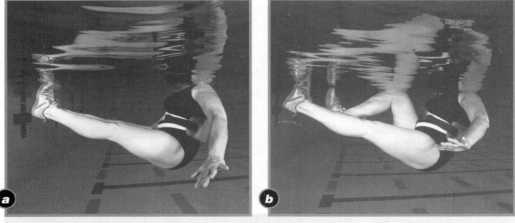

FIGURE 5.49 **Single-leg stretch (Pilates): *(a)* Begin in the V position; *(b)* pull one knee to chest.**

▶ **CUEING TIP:** Begin in V position, pull one knee to chest and return to V.

Double-leg stretch (Pilates); *muscles used:* hip flexors, abdominals stabilize

▶ **CUEING TIP:** Begin in V position, pull both knees to chest and return to V.

Hip curl, travel forward; *muscles used:* hip flexors, abdominals stabilize

▶ **CUEING TIP:** Clap hands; emphasize arms moving away from knees.

Hip curl, travel backward; *muscles used:* hip flexors, abdominals stabilize

▶ **CUEING TIP:** Clap hands; emphasize arms moving toward knees.

Seated leg lift, hold for 15 seconds (see figure 5.50); *muscles used:* hip flexors, abdominals stabilize

▶ **CUEING TIP:** Lift both legs and hold for 15 seconds.

Seated leg lift with one foot on top of the other; *muscles used:* hip flexors, abdominals stabilize

Teaser (Pilates); *muscles used:* hip flexors, abdominals stabilize

▶ **CUEING TIP:** Alternate hip curl with seated leg lift, one foot on top of the other.

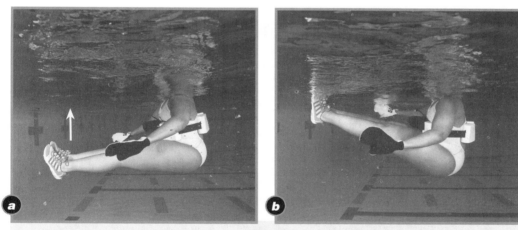

FIGURE 5.50 **Seated leg lift, hold for 15 seconds: *(a)* Begin in the abdominal pike position; *(b)* tighten the abdominals and flex at the hips holding the feet near the surface of the water for 15 seconds.**

OBLIQUES

Lateral rotation; *muscles used:* obliques

Upper-body twist; *muscles used:* obliques

▶ **CUEING TIP:** Jog with hips stable while twisting upper body side to side.

Spine twist (Pilates); *muscles used:* obliques

▶ **CUEING TIP:** Perform upper-body twist slowly in L position with legs wide apart.

Lateral flexion; *muscles used:* obliques

Side crunch from a kneeling position (see figure 5.51); *muscles used:* obliques

▶ **CUEING TIP:** Bring rib cage and pelvis closer together.

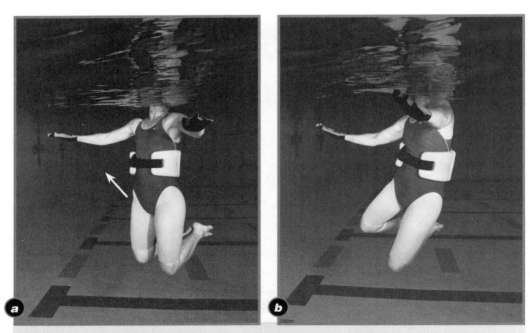

FIGURE 5.51 **Side crunch from a kneeling position:** *(a)* **Begin in a kneeling position;** *(b)* **flex the trunk laterally to bring the rib cage and pelvis closer together.**

Side-to-side extension (see figure 5.52); *muscles used:* obliques

▶ **CUEING TIP:** Extend legs to the side, tuck, and extend legs to the other side.

Side-to-side extension, doubles; *muscles used:* obliques

▶ **CUEING TIP:** Extend legs to the side, tuck and extend again, then tuck and extend legs to the other side 2×.

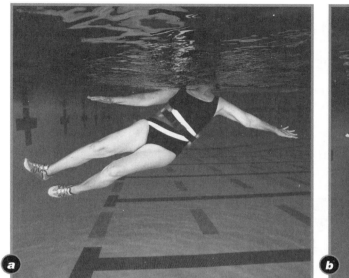

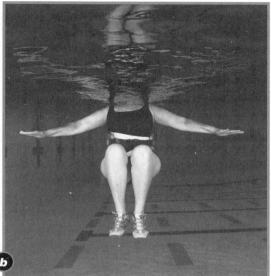

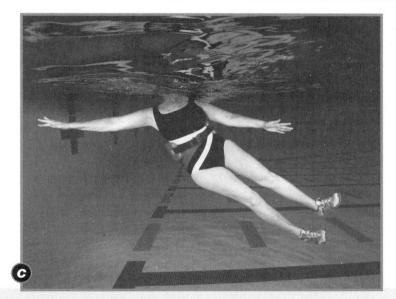

FIGURE 5.52 **Side-to-side extension:** *(a)* **Begin in a side-lying position;** *(b)* **tuck the feet under the body;** *(c)* **extend the legs to the opposite side.**

Side-to-side extension with legs in a diamond position (see figure 5.53); *muscles used:* obliques

▶ **CUEING TIP:** Maintain the diamond position throughout the move.

Side-to-side extension, upper leg or lower leg only; *muscles used:* obliques

Side-to-side extension, R leg or L leg only; *muscles used:* obliques

Side-to-side extension, travel forward; *muscles used:* obliques

▶ **CUEING TIP:** Travel forward in a zigzag.

Extension forward, R, back, L, and reverse; *muscles used:* rectus abdominis, obliques, erector spinae

Side kick (Pilates); *muscles used:* obliques, hip flexors, gluteus maximus

▶ **CUEING TIP:** In a side-lying position, move only the top leg, forward and back, slowly.

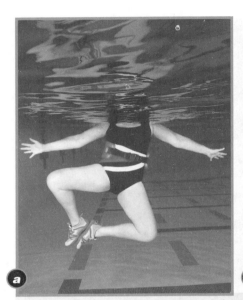
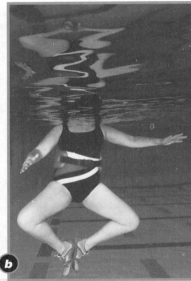
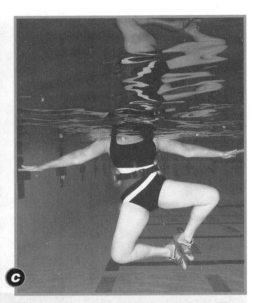

FIGURE 5.53 Side-to-side extension with legs in a diamond position: *(a)* Begin in a side-lying position with the legs in a diamond position; *(b)* bring the diamond under the body; *(c)* continue to the opposite side.

CORE CHALLENGE

Log jump forward and back; *muscles used:* core stabilizers

Log jump, side to side (see figure 5.54); *muscles used:* core stabilizers

▶ **CUEING TIP:** Extend legs 45 degrees to R side, tuck, and extend legs 45 degrees to L side.

Log jump, one side; *muscles used:* core stabilizers

▶ **CUEING TIP:** Extend the legs 45 degrees to one side, tuck, and extend them again to the same side.

Log jump, doubles; *muscles used:* core stabilizers

▶ **CUEING TIP:** Extend legs 45 degrees to the side, tuck and extend again, tuck and extend 45 degrees to the other side 2×.

One leg kicks forward and back (see figure 5.55); *muscles used:* hip flexors, gluteus maximus, core stabilizers

▶ **CUEING TIP:** Keep the other leg stationary.

One leg kicks forward and side; *muscles used:* hip flexors, gluteus medius, core stabilizers

▶ **CUEING TIP:** Keep the other leg stationary.

One leg kicks side and back; *muscles used:* gluteus medius, gluteus maximus, core stabilizers

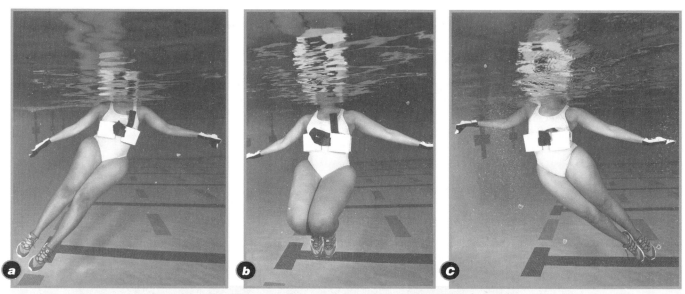

FIGURE 5.54 **Log jump, side to side:** *(a)* **Begin with the legs 45 degrees to one side;** *(b)* **tuck the feet under the body;** *(c)* **extend the legs 45 degrees to the other side.**

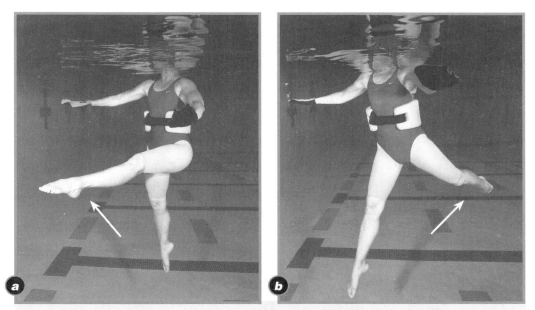

FIGURE 5.55 **One leg kicks forward and back:** *(a)* **Kick one leg forward with the other leg directly under the body;** *(b)* **kick the leg back, keeping the other leg stationary.**

▶ **CUEING TIP:** Keep the other leg stationary.

One leg kicks forward, side, back, side; *muscles used:* hip flexors, gluteus medius, gluteus maximus, core stabilizers

▶ **CUEING TIP:** Keep the other leg stationary.

One leg—knee lift, kick forward, side knee lift, kick side, heel lift, kick back; *muscles used:* hip flexors, gluteus medius, hamstrings, gluteus maximus, core stabilizers

▶ **CUEING TIP:** Keep the other leg stationary.

Straight body with breaststroke (see figure 5.56), reverse breaststroke, or unison sidestroke, travel; *muscles used:* core stabilizers

▶ **CUEING TIP:** Keep ankles crossed.

L position with breaststroke or reverse breaststroke, travel; *muscles used:* core stabilizers

▶ **CUEING TIP:** Keep ankles crossed.

Knees to chest with breaststroke or reverse breaststroke, travel; *muscles used:* core stabilizers

▶ **CUEING TIP:** Keep ankles crossed.

Seated breaststroke (see figure 5.57); *muscles used:* tensor fasciae latae, hip adductors, core stabilizers

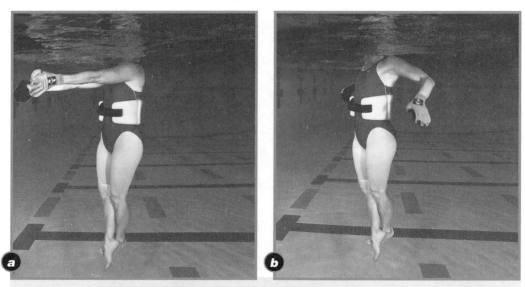

FIGURE 5.56 **Straight body with breaststroke: (a)** Begin in neutral posture with the ankles crossed and the shoulders flexed; **(b)** abduct the arms horizontally in a breaststroke motion maintaining neutral posture.

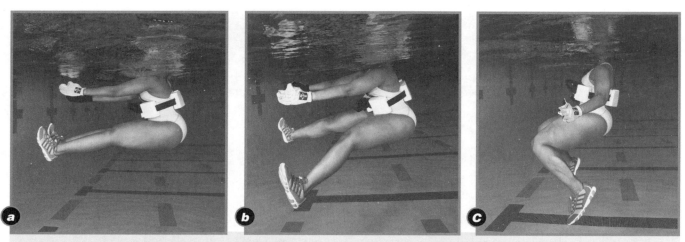

FIGURE 5.57 **Seated breaststroke: (a)** Begin with the hips and shoulders flexed; **(b)** abduct the arms and legs horizontally in a breaststroke motion; **(c)** flex the elbows and knees to return to the starting position.

▶ **CUEING TIP:** Arms and legs do the same thing.

Seated reverse breaststroke; *muscles used:* tensor fasciae latae, hip adductors, core stabilizers

▶ **CUEING TIP:** Arms and legs do the same thing.

Dolphin (see figure 5.58); *muscles used:* core stabilizers

▶ **CUEING TIP:** Undulate the body; travel backward.

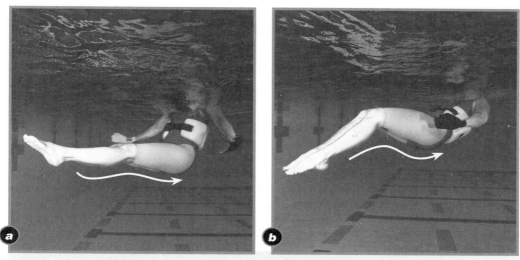

FIGURE 5.58 Dolphin: Extend and flex the hips and knees in a fluid motion.

BALANCE EXERCISES

Standing leg press with one foot on noodle; *muscles used:* core stabilizers, quadriceps, gluteus maximus

Kneel on noodle and balance; *muscles used:* core stabilizers

Kneel on noodle; travel with breaststroke, reverse breaststroke, or sidestroke; *muscles used:* core stabilizers

Stand on noodle and use as a stair climber; *muscles used:* core stabilizers, quadriceps, gluteus maximus

▶ **CUEING TIP:** Lift one knee at a time and press the noodle down with the foot.

Stand on noodle and balance; *muscles used:* core stabilizers

Stand on noodle and balance with one leg lifted forward (see figure 5.59); *muscles used:* core stabilizers

Stand on noodle and balance with one leg extended backward; *muscles used:* core stabilizers

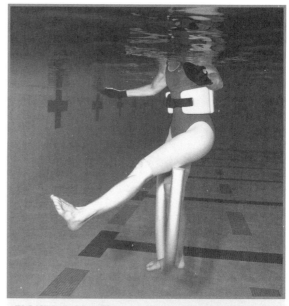

FIGURE 5.59 Stand on noodle and balance with one leg lifted forward: One foot is on the noodle and the other leg is lifted forward.

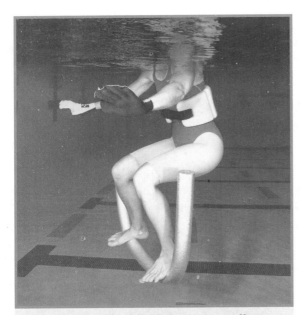

FIGURE 5.60 **Surf: Both feet are on the noodle hip distance apart, hips and knees are flexed.**

Stand on noodle, travel with breaststroke or reverse breaststroke; *muscles used:* core stabilizers

Surf (see figure 5.60); *muscles used:* core stabilizers

▶ **CUEING TIP:** Stand on noodle and pull knees to chest.

Surf, travel with breaststroke, reverse breaststroke, or sidestroke; *muscles used:* core stabilizers

CHAPTER 6

Deep-Water Lesson Plans

Choreography is the way you organize your lesson plan to give it logic and flow and make it easy to remember. This book presents four strategies for developing choreography. They are linear choreography, variations on a theme, add-on choreography, and block choreography.

LINEAR CHOREOGRAPHY

Linear choreography is an easy way to organize a lesson plan. You simply write a list of exercises without repetition, or with very little repetition. Linear choreography can be represented by letters (a, b, c, d, e). Begin with exercise "a" and then go to exercise "b" and so on until you have enough material to fill up your class time. Be sure to include a warm-up, a conditioning phase, and a cool-down. It is helpful to have some kind of theme to your linear choreography so that it doesn't feel like just a random list of exercises. Your theme might be an introduction to basic moves, strength training, a circuit class, deep-water running, traveling, or using noodles.

▶ **Deep-Water Lesson Plan 1**

BASIC MOVES

CLASS OBJECTIVE
Cardiorespiratory fitness

EQUIPMENT
Flotation belt

TEACHING TIP
This class introduces basic moves to new participants, but it also provides experienced participants with a cardiorespiratory workout. Teach from the deck so new participants can see what you are doing. Demonstrate, as well as cue, good posture—*head over shoulders, shoulders over hips, and feet under you.*

WARM-UP
Knee-high jog with jog press

Jacks tuck

Crossover knees

Straddle jog with scull

Run tires with scull

Over the barrel, travel sideways

CONDITIONING PHASE
(A set)

Knee-high jog, scull in front, travel backward

Knee-high jog, scull arms down, travel forward

Knee-high jog with unison sidestroke, travel sideways

Sprint

Heel jog, push forward, travel backward

Heel jog with crawl stroke, travel forward

Cross-country ski, knees bent 90 degrees

Tuck ski

Tuck ski together

Cross-country ski, travel backward and forward

Cross-country ski, diagonal, travel sideways

(B set)

Kick forward with reverse breaststroke, travel backward

Kick forward with breaststroke, travel forward

High kick, travel backward and forward

Cossack kick with sidestroke, travel sideways

Jumping jacks, travel sideways

Jumping jacks, clap hands, travel backward and forward

Jacks cross

Ankle touch

Hopscotch

(C set)

Skate kick with reverse breaststroke, travel backward

Skate kick, hands behind back, travel forward

Flutter kick, scull in front, travel backward

Flutter kick, scull arms down, travel forward

Flutter kick with elevation

Flutter kick, side-lying, travel

Bicycle, side-lying, travel

Bicycle, side-lying, in a circle

Bicycle, diagonal, travel sideways

COOL-DOWN
Seated kick, feet pointed, travel backward

Seated kick, feet flexed, travel forward

Seated reverse breaststroke, travel backward

Seated breaststroke, travel forward

Dolphin, travel backward

Rock climb, travel forward

Crunch, V position

Side crunch from a kneeling position

Seated pelvic tilt

Stretch: hip flexors, quadriceps, gastrocnemius, hamstrings, lower back, shoulders

▶ **Deep-Water Lesson Plan 2**

ARM MOVES, CHANGE LEGS

CLASS OBJECTIVE
Muscular strength and endurance

EQUIPMENT
Flotation belt

TEACHING TIP
Have participants do three sets of 16 repetitions with each upper-body move, but use a different

leg move with each set. Have them shake their arms out and then scull for stability between sets, continuing the leg move for eight repetitions. When they change to the next leg move, they resume the arm moves.

WARM-UP

Instructor's choice

CONDITIONING PHASE

(A set)

Shoulder blade squeeze with knee-high jog

Shoulder blade squeeze with flutter kick

Shoulder blade squeeze with heel jog

Sprint

(B set)

Clap hands with knee-high jog

Clap hands with straddle jog

Clap hands with jumping jacks

Sprint

(C set)

Pec press, hands together, with knee-high jog

Pec press, hands together, with kick forward

Pec press, hands together, with skate kick

Sprint

(D set)

Arm swing with knee-high jog

Arm swing with kick forward

Arm swing with cross-country ski

Sprint

(E set)

Lat pull-down with knee-high jog

Lat pull-down with jumping jacks

Lat pull-down with high kick

Sprint

(F set)

Arm curl with knee-high jog

Arm curl with straddle jog

Arm curl with run tires

Sprint

(G set)

Triceps extension with knee-high jog

Triceps extension with heel jog

Triceps extension with Cossack kick

Sprint

(H set)

Forearm press with knee-high jog

Forearm press, side-to-side, with cross-country ski

Forearm press with flutter kick

Knee-high jog, scull arms down, travel forward

COOL-DOWN

Flutter kick up to L position and down to upright

Flutter kick, side-lying, travel

Side-to-side extension

Hip curl with one foot on top of the other

Seated leg lift with one foot on top of the other

Teaser (Pilates)

Stretch: upper back, pectorals, shoulders, latissimus dorsi, triceps, gastrocnemius

► **Deep-Water Lesson Plan 3**

LEG MOVES, CHANGE ARMS 1

CLASS OBJECTIVES

Cardiorespiratory fitness and muscular strength and endurance

EQUIPMENT

Flotation belt

TEACHING TIP

If participants keep their legs moving while performing 8 to 12 repetitions of each strength training exercise for the upper body, their heart rates will stay in the lower level of their target heart rates. Adding travel on every third strength training exercise will increase not only the resistance for the upper body but also the heart rate. If you add four sets of intervals to bring them into the upper level of their target heart rates, you will accomplish two objectives in one class. In the lesson plans in this book, the exercises used to bring the heart rate up during interval sessions are labeled *interval high intensity phase*. The exercises used to decrease heart rate following the high-intensity phase are labeled *interval active recovery phase*.

WARM-UP

Instructor's choice

CONDITIONING PHASE

(A set)

Knee-high jog with jog press

Knee-high jog with crossovers, emphasize pectorals

Knee-high jog, scull in front and scull arms down, travel backward and forward

Interval high-intensity phase: knee-high jog, faster

Interval active recovery phase: knee-high jog

(B set)

Straddle jog with double-arm press-down

Straddle jog with shoulder blade squeeze

Straddle jog, clap hands, travel backward and forward

(C set)

Run tires, reach to the sides

Run tires with crossovers, emphasize posterior deltoids

Run tires with paddle pull, travel backward and forward

Interval high-intensity phase: run tires with elevation

Interval active recovery phase: run tires

(D set)

Jumping jacks, arms cross in back

Jumping jacks with lat pull-down with elbows bent

Jumping jacks, travel sideways

(E set)

Cross-country ski with windshield wiper arms

Cross-country ski with forearm press, side to side

Cross-country ski with unison arm swing, travel backward and forward

Interval high-intensity phase: cross-country ski with power

Interval active recovery phase: cross-country ski

(F set)

Flutter kick, open and close doors

Flutter kick with lat pull-down

Flutter kick with unison sidestroke, travel sideways

(G set)

Kick forward with triceps press-back

Kick forward with arm lift to sides

Kick forward with reverse breaststroke and breaststroke, travel backward and forward

Interval high-intensity phase: kick forward, faster

Interval active recovery phase: kick forward

(H set)

Heel jog with standing row

Heel jog with hand flutters

Heel jog, push forward and crawl stroke, travel backward and forward

COOL-DOWN

Hip curl, L position

Hip curl with alternating knees

Seated leg lift, hold for 15 seconds

Crunch with legs in a diamond position

Side-to-side extension with legs in a diamond position

Stretch: upper back, pectorals, shoulders, latissimus dorsi, triceps, hip flexors

▶ Deep-Water Lesson Plan 4

LEG MOVES, CHANGE ARMS 2

CLASS OBJECTIVES

Cardiorespiratory fitness and muscular strength and endurance

EQUIPMENT

Flotation belt

TEACHING TIP

Have participants keep their legs moving while they perform 8 to 12 repetitions of each strength training exercise for the upper body. After three sets of strength training exercises, they do a set of intervals to bring them into the upper level of their target heart rates.

WARM-UP

Instructor's choice

CONDITIONING PHASE

(A set)

Cross-country ski

Cross-country ski, push forward

Cross-country ski with unison arm swing

Interval high-intensity phase: cross-country ski, full ROM

Interval active recovery phase: cross-country ski

(B set)

Jumping jacks

Jumping jacks, palms touch in front and in back

Jumping jacks, clap hands

Interval high-intensity phase: mini jacks, faster

Interval active recovery phase: jumping jacks

(C set)

Kick forward with arm swing, palms face direction of motion

Kick forward, elbows together

Kick forward with jump rope arms

Interval high-intensity phase: high kick

Interval active recovery phase: kick forward

(D set)

Skate kick with pumping arms

Skate kick, push arm across

Skate kick with paddlewheel

Interval high-intensity phase: skate kick with power

Interval active recovery phase: skate kick

(E set)

Heel jog with chest fly

Heel jog, open and close doors

Heel jog with hand flutters

Interval high-intensity phase: breaststroke kick with elevation

Interval active recovery phase: heel jog

(F set)

Flutter kick with scull

Flutter kick with reverse breaststroke

Flutter kick with breaststroke

Interval high-intensity phase: flutter kick with elevation

Interval active recovery phase: flutter kick

(G set)

Knee-high jog with standing row

Knee-high jog with arm curl

Knee-high jog with triceps extension

Interval high-intensity phase: steep climb

Interval active recovery phase: knee-high jog

COOL-DOWN

Hip curl from a kneeling position

Side crunch from a kneeling position

Crunch, V position

Side-to-side extension

Side-to-side extension, upper leg only

Side-to-side extension, lower leg only

Stretch: upper back, pectorals, shoulders, latissimus dorsi, triceps, gastrocnemius

► Deep-Water Lesson Plan 5

CIRCUIT WORKOUT 1

CLASS OBJECTIVE

Muscular strength and endurance

EQUIPMENT

Flotation belt

TEACHING TIP

At the end of each set of rhythmic exercises, have participants check their posture before performing the upper-body strength training exercises. Remind them to push hard against the resistance of the water.

WARM-UP

Instructor's choice

CONDITIONING PHASE

(A set)

Knee-high jog with unison arm swing, travel backward and forward

Run tires with alternating paddle pull, travel backward and forward

Seated leg press with unison paddle pull, travel backward and forward

Over the barrel, travel sideways

Straddle jog, palms touch in front

Straddle jog, palms touch in back

(B set)

Jumping jacks, clap hands, travel backward and forward

Jumping jacks, travel sideways

Jacks tuck

Sprint

Knee-high jog with crossovers, emphasize posterior deltoids

Knee-high jog with crossovers, emphasize pectorals

(C set)

Kick forward, push forward and crawl stroke, travel backward and forward

Flutter kick with unison sidestroke, travel sideways

Flutter kick up to L position and down to upright

High kick

Knee-high jog with breaststroke 4× and reverse breaststroke 4×; alternate

(D set)

Cross-country ski, travel backward and forward

Cross-country ski, diagonal, travel sideways

Tuck ski

Cross-country ski with elevation

Knee-high jog with shoulder blade squeeze

Knee-high jog with standing row

(E set)

Seated reverse breaststroke and breaststroke, travel backward and forward

Seated kick, travel backward and forward

Bicycle

Steep climb

Run tires with double-arm press-down

Run tires, push arm across

(F set)

Log jump, side to side

Log jump, one side

Log jump one side, and jacks tuck, alternate

Side-to-side extension

Knee-high jog with arm curl

Knee-high jog, open and close doors

(G set)

One leg kicks forward and back

Abdominal pike and spine extension

Abdominal pike

Mermaid

Knee-high jog with triceps extension

Knee-high jog, push forward

COOL-DOWN

Seated pelvic tilt

Hip curl, L position

Hip curl with alternating knees

The hundred (Pilates)

Rolling like a ball (Pilates)

Stretch: upper back, pectorals, shoulders, latissimus dorsi, triceps, quadriceps

▶ Deep-Water Lesson Plan 6

CIRCUIT WORKOUT 2

CLASS OBJECTIVE

Muscular strength and endurance

EQUIPMENT

Flotation belt

TEACHING TIP

This lesson plan focuses on the muscles on the back of the body, which are used less often than the muscles in front. Cue participants to concentrate on the specific muscle being used. When traveling sideways with jumping jacks, participants may have a tendency to bend the knee to shorten the lever, but this works hamstrings instead of adductors. Remind them to keep the legs straight to work the inner thigh.

WARM-UP

Knee-high jog with jog press

Straddle jog with shoulder blade squeeze

Straddle jog, palms touch in back

Knee-high jog with scull

Knee-high jog, faster, with scull

Knee-high jog, scull in front and scull arms down, travel backward and forward

CONDITIONING PHASE

(A set)

Knee-high jog with breaststroke, travel forward

Knee-high jog with shoulder blade squeeze

Knee-high jog with standing row, travel forward

Knee-high jog, palms touch in back

Knee-high jog with reverse breaststroke, travel backward; sprint, travel in a zigzag

(B set)

High kick, travel forward

Skate kick with pumping arms, travel forward

Cross-country ski, travel forward

One leg kicks forward and back

Knee-high jog, travel in a square and change directions

(C set)

Knee-high jog with triceps press-back, travel forward

Knee-high jog with triceps extension

Knee-high jog, push forward

Knee-high jog with unison jog press

Knee-high jog with quick change of direction

(D set)

Bicycle, travel forward

Heel jog, scull in front and scull arms down, travel backward and forward

Cossack kick with sidestroke, travel sideways

Seated kick, travel forward

Knee-high jog, travel in a circle and reverse

(E set)

Jumping jacks, travel sideways

Jumping jacks, emphasize abduction

Jacks cross

Mini cross

Seated jacks, travel backward and forward

Knee-high jog, travel backward; sprint, travel in a zigzag

Knee-high jog, travel in a square and change directions

Knee-high jog with quick change of direction

Knee-high jog, travel in a circle and reverse

COOL-DOWN

Abdominal pike and spine extension

Abdominal pike and spine extension, legs wide in front and together in back

Abdominal pike and spine extension, legs together in front and wide in back

Abdominal pike and spine extension, legs wide in front and wide in back with tuck in center

Hip curl, V position, travel backward; rock climb, travel forward

Stretch: upper back, lower back, triceps, hamstrings, inner thigh, neck

▶ Deep-Water Lesson Plan 7

CIRCUIT WORKOUT 3

CLASS OBJECTIVE

Muscular strength and endurance

EQUIPMENT

Flotation belt and noodles

TEACHING TIP

Have participants travel for four minutes and then do a strength training exercise for one minute to improve muscular endurance. This lesson plan focuses on the muscles on the back of the body, which are used less often than the muscles in front. The targeted muscles are listed in parentheses after each strength training exercise.

WARM-UP

Knee-high jog with jog press

Straddle jog with scull

Cossack kick

Ankle touch

Hopscotch

Jumping jacks

Jacks tuck

Tuck ski

Cross-country ski

CONDITIONING PHASE

(A set)

Sprint, hands fisted (1 min.)

Sprint, hands cupped (1 min.)

Repeat both

Flutter kick, L position, with crossovers (posterior deltoids) (1 min.)

(B set)

Knee-high jog with breaststroke, travel forward (1 min.)

Knee-high jog with reverse breaststroke, travel backward (1 min.)

Repeat both

Rock climb (gluteus maximus) (1 min.)

(C set)

Knee-high jog with double-arm press-down, travel forward (1 min.)

Knee-high jog, scull in front, travel backward (1 min.)

Repeat both

Tuck knees and lift shoulders out of the water with a triceps extension (triceps) (1 min.)

(D set)

Knee-high jog with crawl stroke, travel forward (1 min.)

Knee-high jog, push forward, travel backward (1 min.)

Repeat both

Seated kick, travel forward (hamstrings) (1 min.)

(E set)

Sprint with resistor arms (1 min.)

Sprint with breaststroke (1 min.)

Repeat both

Lat pull-down, seated jacks position (latissimus dorsi) (1 min.)

(F set)

Sprint, hands cupped (1 min.)

Knee-high jog, hands fisted (1 min.)

Repeat both

Seated jacks, travel backward (adductors) (30 secs.)

Seated jacks, travel forward (tensor fasciae latae) (30 secs.)

COOL-DOWN

(Kneel on noodle)

Travel backward with reverse breaststroke and forward with breaststroke

Travel sideways with sidestroke

(Stand on noodle)

Balance with one leg lifted forward

Balance with one leg extended backward

Stretch: upper back, lower back, triceps, hamstrings, latissimus dorsi, shoulders

▶ **Deep-Water Lesson Plan 8**

SINGLES AND DOUBLES

CLASS OBJECTIVE

Cardiorespiratory fitness

EQUIPMENT

Flotation belt

TEACHING TIP

Single and double moves are a fun way to challenge coordination.

WARM-UP

Instructor's choice

CONDITIONING PHASE

(A set)

Straddle jog

Diamonds

Knee-high jog

Knee-high jog, doubles

Jump rope

Heel jog

Heel jog, doubles

Breaststroke kick

High kick, travel backward

Skate kick, hands behind back, travel forward

Cross-country ski, travel backward and forward

(B set)

Ankle touch

Ankle touch, doubles

Hopscotch

Hopscotch, doubles

High kick, travel backward

Skate kick, hands behind back, travel forward

Cross-country ski, diagonal, travel sideways

(C set)

Knee-high jog, push forward and unison push forward

Knee-high jog with jog press in front and unison jog press in front

Knee-high jog with jog press at sides and unison jog press at sides

Knee-high jog with alternating arm curl and unison arm curl

Kick forward with arm swing and unison arm swing

Knee-high jog with sidestroke and unison sidestroke, travel sideways

Sprint 2 laps

(D set)

Kick forward

Kick forward, doubles

Tuck ski

Tuck ski, doubles

Jacks tuck

Log jump, side to side

Log jump, side to side, doubles

High kick, travel backward

Skate kick, hands behind back, travel forward

Cross-country ski, travel backward and forward

Cross-country ski, diagonal, travel sideways

COOL-DOWN

Seated kick

Mermaid

Hip curl with alternating knees

Hip curl with unison knees

Seated leg lift, hold for 15 seconds

Side-to-side extension

Side-to-side extension, doubles

Stretch: quadriceps, hamstrings, gastrocnemius, inner thigh, shoulders, upper back

▶ Deep-Water Lesson Plan 9

CORE CHALLENGE

CLASS OBJECTIVE

Core strength

EQUIPMENT

Flotation belt

TEACHING TIP

Good core strength helps maintain good posture. Make sure your participants can maintain neutral alignment while performing the basic moves before challenging them with this lesson plan.

WARM-UP

Instructor's choice

CONDITIONING PHASE

(A set)

High kick, travel backward and forward

Jumping jacks, travel sideways

Skate kick with reverse breaststroke and hands behind back, travel backward and forward

High kick

R leg kicks forward 12×, L leg kicks forward 12×

Jumping jacks

R leg kicks side 12×, L leg kicks side 12×

Skate kick with pumping arms

R leg kicks back 12×, L leg kicks back 12×

High kick, travel backward and forward

Jumping jacks, travel sideways

Skate kick with reverse breaststroke and hands behind back, travel backward and forward

High kick

R leg kicks forward and side 8×, L leg kicks forward and side 8×

Jumping jacks

R leg kicks side and back 8×, L leg kicks side and back 8×

Skate kick with pumping arms

R leg kicks forward and back 8×, L leg kicks forward and back 8×

High kick, travel backward and forward

Jumping jacks, travel sideways

Skate kick with reverse breaststroke and hands behind back, travel backward and forward

(B set)

Cross-country ski

Cross-country ski with elevation

Tuck ski

Jacks tuck

Tuck ski and jacks tuck, alternate

Cross-country ski with elevation

Cross-country ski

(C set)

Knee-high jog with reverse breaststroke and breaststroke, travel backward and forward

Straight body with reverse breaststroke and breaststroke, travel backward and forward

Sprint

Knee-high jog with sidestroke, travel sideways

Straight body with unison sidestroke, travel sideways

Sprint

(D set)

Jump rope, travel backward and forward

Log jump, forward and back

Log jump, side to side

Jacks tuck

Log jump one side, and jacks tuck, alternate

Log jump, one side

COOL-DOWN

Abdominal pike and spine extension

Side-to-side extension

Extension forward, R, back, L, and reverse

Abdominal pike

Mermaid

L position with reverse breaststroke and breaststroke, travel backward and forward

Hip curl with one foot on top of the other

Seated leg lift with one foot on top of the other

Teaser (Pilates)

Stretch: lower back, obliques, shoulders, hip flexors, gastrocnemius, neck

► Deep-Water Lesson Plan 10

DEEP-WATER RUNNING

CLASS OBJECTIVE

Cardiorespiratory fitness

EQUIPMENT

Flotation belt

TEACHING TIP

This is a good class for both beginners and experienced deep-water participants. Beginners may not have enough strength to travel with other exercises, but they can be successful with running because it is such a familiar movement. Watch for participants leaning forward, and cue for good posture often. Have them take a break from running and do cross-country ski and jumping jacks occasionally to stretch the muscles in a different direction. If you have enough room, have them run around the perimeter of the pool area as if they were on a running track.

WARM-UP

Instructor's choice

CONDITIONING PHASE

(A set)

Knee-high jog, scull arms down, travel forward

Knee-high jog with crawl stroke, travel forward

Knee-high jog with breaststroke, travel forward

Sprint

Sprint with resistor arms

Sprint with breaststroke

Sprint, hands up

Sprint

Cross-country ski

(B set)

Knee-high jog, scull in front, travel backward

Knee-high jog, push forward, travel backward

Knee-high jog with reverse breaststroke, travel backward

Jumping jacks

(C set)

Knee-high jog with double-arm press-down, travel forward

Knee-high jog with standing row, travel forward

Knee-high jog with breaststroke, travel forward

Sprint

Sprint with resistor arms

Sprint with breaststroke

Sprint, hands up

Sprint

Cross-country ski

(D set)

Knee-high jog, scull in front, travel backward

Knee-high jog, push forward, travel backward

Knee-high jog with reverse breaststroke, travel backward

Jumping jacks

(E set)

Knee-high jog, diagonal, travel sideways

Knee-high jog with unison sidestroke, travel sideways

Cross-country ski, diagonal, travel sideways

Jumping jacks, travel sideways

Bicycle, diagonal, travel sideways

Over the barrel, travel sideways

Cossack kick, travel sideways

COOL-DOWN

Tuck ski together, side-lying, travel

Bicycle, side-lying, travel

Straight body with reverse breaststroke and breaststroke, travel backward and forward

Straight body with unison sidestroke, travel sideways

One leg kicks forward, side, back, side

Stretch: gastrocnemius, quadriceps, hip flexors, hamstrings, outer thigh, shoulders

▶ **Deep-Water Lesson Plan 11**

TRAVEL

CLASS OBJECTIVES

Cardiorespiratory fitness and muscular strength and endurance

EQUIPMENT

Flotation belt

TEACHING TIP

Travel in deep water requires upper-body strength, but it is also a learned skill. Participants have to know when to push or pull hard against the water and when to slice to get the body moving in the desired direction. Position your beginners in the front of the class so you can give them additional coaching while experienced participants travel toward the back of the pool.

WARM-UP

Instructor's choice

CONDITIONING PHASE

(A set)

Knee-high jog, push forward and crawl stroke, travel backward and forward

Knee-high jog with side arm curl, travel sideways

Sprint

(B set)

Flutter kick with reverse breaststroke and breaststroke, travel backward and forward

Flutter kick with unison sidestroke, travel sideways

Flutter kick with elevation

Kick forward with unison arm swing, travel backward and forward

High kick, travel backward and forward

Skate kick with reverse breaststroke and hands behind back, travel backward and forward

(C set)

Cross-country ski, travel backward and forward

Cross-country ski, diagonal, travel sideways

Cross-country ski with elevation

Jumping jacks, clap hands, travel backward and forward

Jumping jacks, travel sideways

Jacks cross

(D set)

Bicycle, scull in front and scull arms down, travel backward and forward

Bicycle, climb a hill

Bicycle, side-lying, travel

Tuck ski together, side-lying, travel

Cross-country ski, side-lying, travel

Seated kick, travel backward and forward

Seated reverse breaststroke and breaststroke, travel backward and forward

COOL-DOWN

Hip curl, V position, travel backward and forward

Dolphin, travel backward; rock climb, travel forward

Log jump, forward and back

Abdominal pike and spine extension

Crunch, V position

Eight short crunches and two long crunches

Log jump, side to side

Stretch: quadriceps, gastrocnemius, hamstrings, outer thigh, inner thigh, obliques

▶ **Deep-Water Lesson Plan 12**

TRAVEL WITH INTERVALS

CLASS OBJECTIVES
Cardiorespiratory fitness and muscular strength and endurance

EQUIPMENT
Flotation belt

TEACHING TIP
The effort required to travel in deep water not only improves muscular strength and endurance, but also offers the potential for burning extra calories. Interval training improves cardiorespiratory fitness. Combining travel with intervals creates a good class for participants who are trying to lose weight.

WARM-UP
Knee-high jog with jog press
Straddle jog with scull
Cossack kick
Run tires, reach to the sides
Jacks tuck
Flutter kick with scull
Bicycle, palms touch in back

CONDITIONING PHASE
(A set)
Knee-high jog, scull in front and scull arms down, travel backward and forward
Knee-high jog with unison arm swing, travel backward and forward
Knee-high jog with unison paddle pull, travel backward and forward
Knee-high jog with forearm press, travel backward and forward
Interval high-intensity phase: cross-country ski, faster
Interval active recovery phase: cross-country ski
Interval high-intensity phase: bicycle, faster
Interval active recovery phase: bicycle
Interval high-intensity phase: mini ski, faster
Interval active recovery phase: cross-country ski

(B set)
Sprint, hands fisted and cupped
Sprint, hands up and hands behind back

Sprint with resistor arms and sprint, travel in a zigzag
Interval high-intensity phase: cross-country ski, full ROM
Interval active recovery phase: cross-country ski
Interval high-intensity phase: jacks cross, full ROM
Interval active recovery phase: jumping jacks
Interval high-intensity phase: high kick
Interval active recovery phase: kick forward

(C set)
Cross-country ski, travel backward and forward
Jumping jacks, clap hands, travel backward and forward
High kick, travel backward; skate kick, travel forward
Jumping jacks, travel sideways
Interval high-intensity phase: cross-country ski with elevation
Interval active recovery phase: cross-country ski
Interval high-intensity phase: flutter kick with elevation
Interval active recovery phase: flutter kick
Interval high-intensity phase: run tires with elevation
Interval active recovery phase: run tires

(D set)
Cross-country ski, diagonal, travel sideways
Bicycle, diagonal, travel sideways
Knee-high jog with single-arm sweep, travel sideways
Knee-high jog with unison sidestroke, travel sideways
Interval high-intensity phase: cross-country ski with power
Interval active recovery phase: cross-country ski
Interval high-intensity phase: steep climb
Interval active recovery phase: knee-high jog
Interval high-intensity phase: bicycle, climb a hill
Interval active recovery phase: bicycle

COOL-DOWN
Seated kick, travel backward and forward
Seated jacks, travel backward and forward

Seated reverse breaststroke and breaststroke, travel backward and forward

Hip curl from a kneeling position

Side crunch from a kneeling position

Side-to-side extension

Side-to-side extension, doubles

V-sit

Hold V and scull to travel forward

Stretch: shoulders, upper back, pectorals, quadriceps, hamstrings, inner thigh, outer thigh

▶ **Deep-Water Lesson Plan 13**

TRAVEL UPRIGHT AND SEATED 1

CLASS OBJECTIVES

Cardiorespiratory fitness and muscular strength and endurance

EQUIPMENT

Flotation belt

TEACHING TIP

To experience improvements in cardiorespiratory fitness as well as muscular strength and endurance, your participants need to put effort into the more intense segments of the class. If they are traveling around the perimeter of the pool area, reserve a section in the middle of the pool where those who are unable to work with that kind of intensity can perform the exercises at a slower pace.

WARM-UP

Knee-high jog with jog press

Straddle jog with shoulder blade squeeze

Seated kick, palms touch in back

Bicycle

Bicycle, tandem

Bicycle, diagonal, travel sideways

Bicycle, side-lying, travel

CONDITIONING PHASE

(A set) (intensity level 1)

Knee-high jog, hands fisted, travel forward (1 min.)

Knee-high jog, scull in front, travel backward (1 min.)

Kick forward with unison arm swing, travel forward (1 min.)

Jumping jacks, clap hands, travel backward (1 min.)

Knee-high jog, hands cupped, travel forward (1 min.)

Flutter kick, L position, scull in front, travel backward (1 min.)

Seated kick with unison arm swing, travel forward (1 min.)

Seated jacks, travel backward (1 min.)

(B set) (intensity level 2)

Knee-high jog with breaststroke, travel forward (1 min.)

Straddle jog, clap hands, travel backward (1 min.)

Seated breaststroke, travel forward (1 min.)

Seated leg press, travel backward (1 min.)

Bicycle, tandem with power, travel forward (1 min.)

Knee-high jog with reverse breaststroke, travel backward (1 min.)

Bicycle, tandem with power, travel forward (1 min.)

Seated reverse breaststroke, travel backward (1 min.)

Cross-country ski, travel forward (1 min.)

Knee-high jog, push forward, travel backward (1 min.)

Cross-country ski, travel forward (1 min.)

Jump rope, travel backward (1 min.)

Jumping jacks, clap hands, travel forward (1 min.)

High kick, travel backward (1 min.)

Seated jacks, travel forward (1 min.)

Dolphin, travel backward (1 min.)

(C set) (intensity level 1)

Knee-high jog, hands fisted, travel forward (1 min.)

Knee-high jog, scull in front, travel backward (1 min.)

Kick forward with unison arm swing, travel forward (1 min.)

Jumping jacks, clap hands, travel backward (1 min.)

Knee-high jog, hands cupped, travel forward (1 min.)

Flutter kick, L position, scull in front, travel backward (1 min.)

Seated kick with unison arm swing, travel forward (1 min.)

Seated jacks, travel backward (1 min.)

COOL-DOWN

Cross-country ski, side-lying, travel

Bicycle, side-lying, travel

Bicycle, side-lying, in a circle

Side-to-side extension

Seated leg lift, hold for 15 seconds

Crunch with legs in a diamond position

Stretch: gastrocnemius, quadriceps, hamstrings, outer thigh, hip flexors, shoulders

▶ Deep-Water Lesson Plan 14

TRAVEL UPRIGHT AND SEATED 2

CLASS OBJECTIVES

Cardiorespiratory fitness and muscular strength and endurance

EQUIPMENT

Flotation belt and noodles

TEACHING TIP

By using a variety of arm and leg movements while traveling in deep water, participants can get the benefits of cardio and strength training in a single class. Have them continue the strength training using noodles for resistance during the cool-down segment of the class. They can also use the noodles for balance training.

WARM-UP

Instructor's choice

CONDITIONING PHASE

(A set)

Kick forward, scull in front and scull arms down, travel backward and forward

Kick forward with sidestroke, travel sideways

Seated kick, feet pointed, travel backward

Heel jog, push forward and crawl stroke, travel backward and forward

Heel jog, diagonal, travel sideways

Seated kick, feet flexed, travel forward

Sprint

(B set)

Flutter kick with reverse breaststroke and breaststroke, travel backward and forward

Flutter kick with unison sidestroke, travel sideways

Seated flutter kick, no hands and with unison arm swing, travel backward and forward

Cross-country ski, travel backward and forward

Cross-country ski, diagonal, travel sideways

High kick, travel backward and forward

Sprint

(C set)

Jumping jacks, clap hands, travel backward and forward

Jumping jacks, travel sideways

Seated jacks, travel backward and forward

Straddle jog with alternating paddle pull, travel backward and forward

Straddle jog with single-arm sweep, travel sideways

Seated leg press with unison paddle pull, travel backward and forward

Sprint

(D set)

Bicycle with unison arm swing, travel backward and forward

Bicycle, diagonal, travel sideways

Bicycle, side-lying, travel

COOL-DOWN

(Noodle in hands)

Knee-high jog with standing row

Straddle jog, push noodle down in front

Knee-high jog, push noodle down on one side

Jumping jacks, touch ends of noodle in front

Straddle jog with double-arm press-down, hold ends of noodle together

Jumping jacks, touch ends of noodle in back

Knee-high jog with forearm press, noodle around waist

(Kneel on noodle)

Travel backward with reverse breaststroke and forward with breaststroke

Travel sideways with sidestroke

Stretch: upper back, pectorals, latissimus dorsi, triceps, shoulders, quadriceps, hamstrings

▶ **Deep-Water Lesson Plan 15**

ALL-NOODLE WORKOUT

CLASS OBJECTIVE
Muscular strength and endurance

EQUIPMENT
Flotation belt and noodles

TEACHING TIP
Spice up your class occasionally with an all-noodle workout. The partner moves add fun.

WARM-UP
(Hold noodle in hands)
Knee-high jog
Straddle jog
Cossack kick
Jacks tuck
Jumping jacks
Flutter kick
Kick forward
Heel jog

CONDITIONING PHASE
(A set)
Knee-high jog, push noodle forward
Knee-high jog with standing row
Knee-high jog, diagonal, noodle under arm, travel sideways
Knee-high jog with lat pull-down, noodle in one hand, travel sideways
Jumping jacks, touch ends of noodle in front
Push-ups
Cross-country ski, noodle in R hand, travel sideways
Sprint, hold noodle up
Cross-country ski, noodle in L hand, travel sideways
Sprint, hold noodle up
Jumping jacks, touch ends of noodle in front
Push-ups
Cross-country ski, diagonal, noodle under arm, travel sideways
Knee-high jog with double-arm lift, travel backward
Knee-high jog with double-arm press-down, travel forward

Jumping jacks with forearm press, noodle around waist

(B set) (Straddle noodle)
High kick
Ankle touch
Bicycle reverse, travel backward; bicycle, tandem, travel forward
Seated reverse breaststroke and breaststroke, travel backward and forward

(C set) (Noodle behind shoulders)
Cross-country ski, side-lying, travel
Tuck ski together, side-lying, travel
Knee-high jog, side-lying, travel
Bicycle, side-lying, travel

(D set)
Partner cross-country ski (partners hold opposite ends of two noodles)
Partner jumping jacks
Partner ski–jacks combo (cue: *ski, ski, jack, together*)
Tug of war (partners back to back, hold ends of both noodles under arms and run in opposite directions)
Partner bicycle in a circle (partners back to back, noodles behind shoulders and linked)
Bicycle races (partner 1 runs with noodle in front and under arms; partner 2 straddles a noodle and bicycles holding ends of partner 1's noodle)
Rickshaw (partner 1 runs holding ends of noodles under arms; partner 2 floats in a seated position holding opposite ends)
Canoe races (straddle noodle and paddle with arms)

COOL-DOWN
(Noodle under chest)
Rock climb
(Noodle in hands)
Abdominal pike and spine extension
Side-to-side extension
(Stand on noodle)
Standing leg press with one foot on noodle
Use as a stair climber
Surf

Balance with one leg lifted forward

Balance with one leg extended backward

Stretch: upper back, pectorals, obliques, triceps, gastrocnemius, hip flexors, outer thigh

VARIATIONS ON A THEME

Variations on a theme is a type of linear choreography. Instead of using many different exercises, though, you limit yourself to two or three basic exercises and work these through multiple variations. The choreography can be represented by the letters a1, a2, a3, b1, b2, b3. For example, in Deep-Water Lesson Plan 16, "a" is knee-high jog and "b" is run tires, and the numbers 1, 2, 3 are the variations:

a. Knee-high jog, with 1. Upper-body twist

a. Knee-high jog, with 2. Speed (faster)

a. Knee-high jog, with 3. Chest fly

a. Knee-high jog, with 4. Power (Steep climb)

b. Run tires, with 1. Reach to the sides

b. Run tires, with 2. Speed (faster)

If you would like to try writing your own variations on a theme, begin by selecting your basic exercises. You want to use exercises that work different muscle groups to avoid the fatigue that would come from using a single muscle group for an entire class. An example is to use cross-country ski, which works the legs front to back, and jumping jacks, which work the legs to the sides. What arm moves can you add to the leg moves? Some arm moves can slice, reducing resistance, and some can have the palms face the direction of motion to increase resistance. Try changing the working positions from upright to diagonal to side-lying to seated. Have participants travel forward, backward, or sideways in the various working positions. Add intensity by increasing speed, range of motion, or power, or decrease intensity by having participants slow down, make the move smaller, or back off from pushing hard against the water. Can you change the move to cross the midline of the body, or combine it with another move? Thinking about all the ways to change an exercise will help you come up with your own variations on a theme.

▶ **Deep-Water Lesson Plan 16**

KNEE AND HEEL

CLASS OBJECTIVE

Cardiorespiratory fitness

EQUIPMENT

Flotation belt

TEACHING TIP

Raising the hands up in deep water makes the body sink and forces the legs to work harder. Raising the arms overhead, however, stimulates the pressor response and raises the heart rate. Limit the length of time your participants work with the hands overhead to 15 to 30 seconds, or cue raising the hands to just above the ears. Participants with high blood pressure should not raise their hands above their heads (YMCA, 2000).

WARM-UP

Knee-high jog with jog press

Knee-high jog with shoulder blade squeeze

Run tires with scull

Run tires, reach to the sides

Heel jog, palms touch in back

Heel jog with triceps extension

Tuck ski

Tuck ski together

CONDITIONING PHASE

(A set)

Knee-high jog with upper-body twist

Knee-high jog, faster

Knee-high jog with chest fly

Steep climb

Run tires, reach to the sides

Run tires, faster

Heel jog with arm curl

Heel jog, faster

Tuck ski together

Tuck ski together, faster

(B set)

Knee-high jog

Knee-high jog, diagonal, travel sideways

Knee-high jog, hands up

Knee-high jog with elevation

Run tires

Seated leg press with unison paddle pull, travel backward and forward

Run tires, hands up

Run tires with elevation

Heel jog

Heel jog, diagonal, travel sideways

Heel jog, hands up

Heel jog with elevation

(C set)

Knee-high jog

Knee-high jog, one knee only, with sidestroke, travel sideways

Ankle touch

Run tires

In in, out out

Heel jog

Heel jog, one heel only, with sidestroke, travel sideways

Hopscotch

Ankle touch and hopscotch, alternate

Ankle touch and hopscotch, one side only

(D set)

Knee-high jog, scull in front and scull arms down, travel backward and forward

Sprint

Run tires with sidestroke, travel sideways

Over the barrel, travel sideways

Run tires with paddle pull, travel backward and forward

Heel jog, push forward and crawl stroke, travel backward and forward

Ankle touch, travel backward

Hopscotch, travel forward

Tuck ski together, side-lying, travel

COOL-DOWN

Bicycle, side-lying travel

Bicycle, side-lying, in a circle

Bicycle

Bicycle, one leg only

Bicycle, reverse, travel backward; bicycle, tandem, travel forward

Abdominal pike and spine extension

Stretch: hip flexors, quadriceps, gastrocnemius, hamstrings, lower back, shoulders

► Deep-Water Lesson Plan 17

CROSS-COUNTRY SKI AND JUMPING JACKS

CLASS OBJECTIVE

Cardiorespiratory fitness

EQUIPMENT

Flotation belt

TEACHING TIP

When your class focuses on variations of two exercises, be sure that participants stretch the muscle groups used in those two exercises at the end of the cool-down.

WARM-UP

Instructor's choice

CONDITIONING PHASE

(A set)

Cross-country ski, knees bent 90 degrees

Cross-country ski

Cross-country ski, clap hands

Cross-country ski with unison arm swing

Cross-country ski with forearm press, side to side

Cross-country ski, faster

Jumping jacks

Jumping jacks, arms cross in front

Jumping jacks, arms cross in back

Jumping jacks, arms cross in front and back, alternate

Jumping jacks, faster

(B set)

Cross-country ski, diagonal, travel sideways

Cross-country ski, side-lying, travel

Tuck ski together

Tuck ski together, side-lying, travel

Cross-country ski with elevation

Jumping jacks

Jumping jacks, side-lying

Jumping jacks, 45 degrees

Seated jacks, travel backward and forward

(C set)
Mini ski
Cross-country ski, full ROM
Mini jacks
Jacks cross, full ROM
Mini cross
Triple crossover

(D set)
Cross-country ski, corner to corner
Tuck ski
Tuck ski, corner to corner
Cross-country ski and jumping jacks, alternate
Jacks tuck
Tuck ski and jacks tuck, alternate

(E set)
Cross-country ski; travel backward, forward, and sideways with sidestroke
Cross-country ski with quarter turn
Cross-country ski 3 1/2×, half turn
Jumping jacks, clap hands, travel backward and forward
Jumping jacks, travel sideways
Jumping jacks with quarter turn
Jacks cross 3 1/2×, half turn

COOL-DOWN
Seated Cossack kick
Seated Cossack kick with alternating legs
Cossack kick, diagonal
Flutter kick, side-lying
Side kick (Pilates)
Single-leg stretch (Pilates)
Double-leg stretch (Pilates)
Stretch: hamstrings, outer thigh, inner thigh, hip flexors, gastrocnemius, latissimus dorsi

▶ Deep-Water Lesson Plan 18

<u>KICKS</u>

CLASS OBJECTIVE
Cardiorespiratory fitness

EQUIPMENT
Flotation belt

TEACHING TIP
Some participants tend to power pop the knees when kicking, which is hard on the knee joint. Cue soft knees.

WARM-UP
Kick forward with scull
Kick forward with arm swing
Seated kick
Cossack kick
Skate kick with hands on hips
Skate kick with pumping arms
Flutter kick with arms extended to sides

CONDITIONING PHASE

(A set)
Kick forward, clap hands
Kick forward, faster
Cossack kick with shoulder blade squeeze
Cossack kick, faster
Skate kick, push forward
Skate kick, faster
Flutter kick, feet pointed and flexed
Flutter kick with lat pull-down
Flutter kick, faster

(B set)
Seated kick, travel backward and forward
Mermaid
Seated Cossack kick
Cossack kick, diagonal, travel sideways
Flutter kick, diagonal, travel sideways
Flutter kick, side-lying, travel
Flutter kick, hands up

(C set)
High kick
Skate kick, higher
Flutter kick with elevation
High kick, power down
Skate kick with power

(D set)
Kick forward with reverse breaststroke and breaststroke, travel backward and forward
High kick, travel backward and forward
Cossack kick with sidestroke, travel sideways

Skate kick with reverse breaststroke and hands behind back, travel backward and forward

Flutter kick with unison sidestroke, travel sideways

(E set)

One leg kicks forward

One leg kicks back

One leg kicks forward and back

One leg kicks forward, side, back, side

One leg—knee lift, kick forward, side knee lift, kick side, heel lift, kick back

Kick forward

Kick to the corners

Kick forward and kick to the corners, alternate

COOL-DOWN

Seated flutter kick, scull in front and scull arms down, travel backward and forward

Seated bicycle with reverse breaststroke and breaststroke, travel backward and forward

Seated jacks, travel backward and forward

Dolphin, travel backward; side-to-side extension, travel forward

Stretch: hip flexors, quadriceps, outer thigh, inner thigh, hamstrings, lower back

▶ **Deep-Water Lesson Plan 19**

JOG AND LOG JUMP

CLASS OBJECTIVE

Cardiorespiratory fitness

EQUIPMENT

Flotation belt

TEACHING TIP

Try several different cues for good posture to get the idea across (e.g., *Ears over shoulders, shoulders over hips, feet under you; Chest up, shoulders back; Tuck the chin in; Jog as if you had a book on your head*). For the arm medley, choose any upper-body moves you like.

WARM-UP

Knee-high jog

Straddle jog

Jacks tuck

Log jump, side to side

Side-to-side extension

Knee-high jog, scull in front and scull arms down, travel backward and forward

CONDITIONING PHASE

(A set)

Knee-high jog

Knee-high jog, faster

Steep climb

Straddle jog

Straddle jog, faster

Log jump, forward and back

Abdominal pike and spine extension

(B set)

Knee-high jog with upper-body twist

Knee-high jog with arm medley

Sprint

(C set)

Knee-high jog with sidestroke, travel sideways

Knee-high jog, diagonal, travel sideways

Knee-high jog, side-lying, travel

Knee-high jog, hands up, travel forward

Knee-high jog with elevation

Straddle jog with sidestroke, travel sideways

Straddle jog, diagonal, travel sideways

Straddle jog, hands up, travel forward

Straddle jog with elevation

Frog kick with elevation

Ankle touch, travel backward

Hopscotch, travel forward

Log jump, one side

Side-to-side extension, upper leg only

Side-to-side extension, lower leg only

(D set)

Knee-high jog

Knee-high jog, one knee only, with sidestroke, travel sideways

Straddle jog

Cossack kick

Diamonds

Side-to-side extension with legs in a diamond position

Cossack kick with sidestroke, travel sideways

COOL-DOWN

Seated leg press, travel backward; seated kick, travel forward

Dolphin, travel backward; side-to-side extension, travel forward

Crunch, V position

Seated Cossack kick

Seated jacks, toes in

Seated jacks, toes out

Stretch: hip flexors, quadriceps, hamstrings, outer thigh, obliques, upper back, neck

▶ **Deep-Water Lesson Plan 20**

BICYCLE, CROSS-COUNTRY SKI, AND JUMPING JACKS

CLASS OBJECTIVE

Cardiorespiratory fitness

EQUIPMENT

Flotation belt

TEACHING TIP

Some participants have a tendency to turn toward the direction they want to travel on diagonal moves, which twists their spines out of neutral. Be sure to cue keeping the shoulders and hips squared.

WARM-UP

Bicycle with scull

Cross-country ski, knees bent 90 degrees

Jumping jacks with arms extended to sides

Bicycle with scull

Tuck ski

Jacks tuck

Bicycle, scull in front and scull arms down, travel backward and forward

CONDITIONING PHASE

(A set)

Bicycle with crossovers, palms down

Bicycle, clap hands

Bicycle, faster

Cross-country ski, hands slicing

Cross-country ski, palms face direction of motion

Cross-country ski, faster

Jumping jacks, arms cross in front and in back

Jumping jacks, palms touch in front and in back

Jumping jacks, faster

(B set)

Bicycle, diagonal, travel sideways

Bicycle, side-lying, travel

Bicycle, side-lying, in a circle and reverse

Bicycle with elevation

Cross-country ski, diagonal, travel sideways

Cross-country ski, side-lying, travel

Cross-country ski with elevation

Jumping jacks, side-lying

Seated jacks, travel backward and forward

(C set)

Bicycle, climb a hill

Cross-country ski with power

Jumping jacks with power

(D set)

Seated bicycle

Seated kick

Crossover kick

Cross-country ski, corner to corner

Skate kick

Jacks cross

Mini cross

Triple crossover

Ankle touch

Ankle touch, one ankle only

Hopscotch

Hopscotch, one heel only

(E set)

Bicycle, reverse, travel backward

Bicycle, tandem, travel forward

Cross-country ski; travel backward, forward, and sideways with unison sidestroke

Jumping jacks, clap hands, travel backward and forward

Jumping jacks, travel sideways

COOL-DOWN

Diamonds, upright and seated, alternate

Hip curl with legs in a diamond position

Crunch with legs in a diamond position

Side-to-side extension with legs in a diamond position

Abdominal pike and spine extension with legs in a diamond position

Stretch: hamstrings, inner thigh, outer thigh, quadriceps, hip flexors, gastrocnemius

ADD-ON CHOREOGRAPHY

Add-on choreography is another type of choreography that is easy to write. It is called "add-on" because after you teach a set of exercises, you add on a second set. Repeat those two sets and then add on a third set. Continue the pattern, adding a new set each time around. Add-on choreography can be represented by the letters AB, ABC, ABCD, and so on. You will need five to seven sets of exercises with four to six exercises in each set for a typical class. Select exercises that work well together. The exercises may work well together because they are similar types (e.g., kicks); they all work the body in the same direction (e.g., front to back); or they set up a simple travel pattern (e.g., travel backward with one exercise and forward with another). If you decide to include travel, allow enough time for your participants to move from one end of their area to the other. Use your creativity in putting sets together and you will soon have lots of ideas for add-on choreography.

▶ Deep-Water Lesson Plan 21

ADD-ON CHOREOGRAPHY 1

CLASS OBJECTIVE

Cardiorespiratory fitness

EQUIPMENT

Flotation belt

TEACHING TIP

Have participants perform each exercise 16 times the first time you teach a set; then you can pick up the pace if you like by having them perform the exercises 8 times, or even 4 times, the next time around. When you move on to the next exercise quickly, it is more challenging to keep up.

WARM-UP

Instructor's choice

CONDITIONING PHASE

(A set)

Kick forward

Kick to the corners

Cossack kick

Cross-country ski

(B set)

Kick forward

Skate kick

Seated kick

One leg kicks forward and back

(Repeat A and B sets and add C set)

Ankle touch

Hopscotch

Ankle touch and hopscotch, alternate

(Repeat A-C sets and add D set)

Crossover knees

Crossover kick

High kick 7×, tuck and turn

(Repeat A-D sets and add E set)

Tuck ski together

Cross-country ski

Cross-country ski 3 1/2×, half turn

Mini ski

(Repeat A-E sets and add F set)

Jumping jacks

Jacks cross

Jacks cross 3 1/2×, half turn

Mini jacks

(Repeat A-F sets and add G set)

Knee-high jog

Heel jog

Bicycle

Bicycle, small circles

COOL-DOWN

Mermaid

Seated Cossack kick

Seated jacks

Abdominal pike and spine extension

Abdominal pike and spine extension, legs wide in front and wide in back with tuck in center

Jumping jacks, side-lying

Stretch: quadriceps, gastrocnemius, hamstrings, outer thigh, obliques, shoulders

▶ **Deep-Water Lesson Plan 22**

ADD-ON CHOREOGRAPHY 2

CLASS OBJECTIVES

Cardiorespiratory fitness and muscular strength and endurance

EQUIPMENT

Flotation belt and noodles

TEACHING TIP

Try strength training by having participants use noodles for resistance during the cool-down. Then have them stand on the noodles for balance training.

WARM-UP

Instructor's choice

CONDITIONING PHASE

(A set)

Jumping jacks 4× and turn 4×

Sprint

Cross-country ski, travel backward

Kick forward with crawl stroke, travel forward

(B set)

Seated jacks, travel backward

Over the barrel, travel R

Seated jacks, travel backward

Over the barrel, travel L

(Repeat A and B sets and add C set)

Heel jog, push forward, travel backward

Skate kick, hands behind back, travel forward

(Repeat A-C sets and add D set)

Tuck ski together

R leg kicks forward and back

Cross-country ski with elevation

Repeat set with L leg kicks forward and back

(Repeat A-D sets and add E set)

Jumping jacks, clap hands, travel backward

Sprint, travel in a zigzag

Cross-country ski, travel backward

Sprint, hands up

COOL-DOWN

(Noodle in hands)

Knee-high jog with standing row

Knee-high jog, push noodle forward

Straddle jog, push noodle down in front

Knee-high jog, push noodle down on one side

Straddle jog, touch ends of noodle in front

Straddle jog with double-arm press-down, hold ends of noodle together

Knee-high jog, touch ends of noodle in back

Knee-high jog with forearm press, noodle around waist

(Stand on noodle)

Travel backward with reverse breaststroke and forward with breaststroke

Balance with one leg lifted forward

Balance with one leg extended backward

Surf

Surf, travel backward with reverse breaststroke and forward with breaststroke

Stretch: lower back, hamstrings, outer thigh, upper back, pectorals, triceps, shoulders

▶ **Deep-Water Lesson Plan 23**

ADD-ON CHOREOGRAPHY 3

CLASS OBJECTIVE

Cardiorespiratory fitness

EQUIPMENT

Flotation belt

TEACHING TIP

You can alternate two exercises to increase intensity. Have participants do four repetitions of each pair of exercises in sets C and D, alternating back and forth three times.

WARM-UP

Instructor's choice

CONDITIONING PHASE

(A set)

Jumping jacks, clap hands, travel backward

Cross-country ski, travel forward

Tuck ski together

Seated reverse breaststroke, travel backward

Cross-country ski, travel forward

Tuck ski together

(B set)

Over the barrel, travel R

Sprint

Bicycle, side-lying, circle R

Over the barrel, travel L

Sprint

Bicycle, side-lying, circle L

(Repeat A and B sets and add C set)

Knee-high jog and cross-country ski, corner to corner; alternate 3×

Knee-high jog, faster and tuck ski; alternate 3×

Knee-high jog and high kick 7×, tuck and turn; alternate 3×

Knee-high jog, faster and frog kick; alternate 3×

(Repeat A-C sets and add D set)

Hopscotch and skate kick, alternate 3×

Ankle touch and jacks cross, alternate 3×

Steep climb and bicycle with elevation, alternate 3×

(Repeat A-D sets and add E set)

R leg kicks forward and back, cross-country ski, L leg kicks forward and back

Jacks tuck; log jump, side to side; side-to-side extension

Cross-country ski and jumping jacks, alternate

Kick forward; seated kick, travel backward; high kick, travel forward

COOL-DOWN

Crunch, V position

V-sit

Hold V and scull to travel forward

Cross-country ski, side-lying

Side kick (Pilates)

Stretch: outer thigh, inner thigh, hamstrings, quadriceps, latissimus dorsi, obliques

BLOCK CHOREOGRAPHY

Block choreography is more complex than linear or add-on choreography, but once you get the pattern down, you will be able to come up with many variations. One way to write block choreography is to begin by writing a 10-minute sample class. What will you include? You have many options to choose from such as intervals, travel, upper-body moves, diagonal moves, one-sided moves, doubles, and combining two moves. Your 10-minute sample class is your first set. What can you change for the second set? If you used intervals, can you think of a different way to increase intensity? If you used travel, can you have participants travel in a different direction? If you used upper-body moves, can you think of exercises for a different muscle group? The changes you make to your 10-minute sample class are your second set. Repeat the process two more times, and you have written a 40-minute conditioning set. Block choreography can be represented by the letters a1, b1, c1, d1; a2, b2, c2, d2; a3, b3, c3, d3, and so on. Look, for example, at the two sample sets below. The exercises in the first set are repeated with variations in the second set.

(A set)

(a1) Flutter kick

(b1) Heel jog with shoulder blade squeeze

(c1) Bicycle

(d1) Cross-country ski

(e1) Jumping jacks

(B set)

(a2) Flutter kick with elevation (add elevation)

(b2) Heel jog, clap hands (different arm move)

(c2) Bicycle, travel backward and forward (add travel)

(d2) Cross-country ski, corner to corner (cross midline of body)

(e2) Jacks cross (increase ROM)

You don't have to change everything in your block choreography sets. You may wish to begin each set with the same three exercises, repeat a move from the first set in the third set, or have more sets of fewer exercises. Once you get started, the variations are endless.

▶ **Deep-Water Lesson Plan 24**

UPRIGHT AND SEATED MOVES

CLASS OBJECTIVE
Cardiorespiratory fitness

EQUIPMENT
Flotation belt

TEACHING TIP
The sets begin with cross-country ski and a variation of cross-country ski. Then each set features a different exercise adding an upper-body move, travel, intervals, and travel in a seated position.

WARM-UP
Instructor's choice

CONDITIONING PHASE

(A set)
Cross-country ski, knees bent 90 degrees
Cross-country ski
Kick forward with shoulder blade squeeze
Kick forward with reverse breaststroke and breaststroke, travel backward and forward
Interval high-intensity phase: high kick
Interval active recovery phase: kick forward
Seated kick, no hands and with breaststroke, travel backward and forward

(B set)
Cross-country ski
Cross-country ski, corner to corner
Heel jog with standing row
Heel jog with reverse breaststroke and breaststroke, travel backward and forward
Interval high-intensity phase: breaststroke kick with elevation
Interval active recovery phase: heel jog
Seated kick with reverse breaststroke and no hands, travel backward and forward

(C set)
Cross-country ski
Cross-country ski, full ROM
Flutter kick with lat pull-down

Flutter kick with reverse breaststroke and breaststroke, travel backward and forward
Interval high-intensity phase: mini ski, faster
Interval active recovery phase: flutter kick
Seated flutter kick with reverse breaststroke and breaststroke, travel backward and forward

(D set)
Cross-country ski
Cross-country ski, palms face direction of motion
Jumping jacks with elbows bent
Jumping jacks, clap hands, travel backward and forward
Interval high-intensity phase: mini jacks, faster
Interval active recovery phase: jumping jacks
Seated jacks, travel backward and forward

(E set)
Cross-country ski
Tuck ski together
Knee-high jog with arm curl, palms face direction of motion
Knee-high jog with reverse breaststroke and breaststroke, travel backward and forward
Interval high-intensity phase: steep climb
Interval active recovery phase: knee-high jog
Hip curl, V position, travel backward; and rock climb, travel forward

(F set)
Cross-country ski
Tuck ski, corner to corner
Bicycle with unison jog press
Bicycle with reverse breaststroke and breaststroke, travel backward and forward
Interval high-intensity phase: bicycle, climb a hill
Interval active recovery phase: bicycle

COOL-DOWN
Bicycle, side-lying, travel
Tuck ski together, side-lying, travel
Flutter kick, side-lying, travel
Jumping jacks, side-lying
Side-to-side extension
Stretch: pectorals, upper back, lower back, hamstrings, quadriceps, outer thigh

▶ **Deep-Water Lesson Plan 25**

UPPER BODY AND SPRINTS

CLASS OBJECTIVES

Cardiorespiratory fitness and muscular strength and endurance

EQUIPMENT

Flotation belt

TEACHING TIP

Each set includes upper-body strength training exercises focusing on different muscle groups performed with the legs moving for stability. Finish off the set with sprints the length of the pool to bring participants' heart rates into the upper level of their target heart rates; then use a core challenge exercise for the active recovery.

WARM-UP

Instructor's choice

CONDITIONING PHASE

(A set)
One leg kicks forward and back
High kick
Ankle touch
Knee-high jog with crossovers
Knee-high jog with chest fly
Knee-high jog with shoulder blade squeeze
Knee-high jog with standing row
Straddle jog, clap hands, travel backward and
   forward
Sprint
Straight body with reverse breaststroke and
   breaststroke, travel backward and forward

(B set)
One leg kicks forward and back
Skate kick
Hopscotch
Jumping jacks, palms touch in front
Jumping jacks, palms touch in back
Jumping jacks, palms touch in front and in back
Jumping jacks with elbows bent
Knee-high jog with unison arm swing, travel
   backward and forward

Sprint 2 laps
Straight body with unison sidestroke, travel
   sideways

(C set)
One leg kicks forward and back
High kick
Ankle touch
Knee-high jog, open and close doors
Knee-high jog with arm curl
Knee-high jog with triceps extension
Knee-high jog, push forward and unison jog
   press, travel backward and forward
Sprint 3 laps
L position with reverse breaststroke and breast-
   stroke; travel backward and forward

(D set)
One leg kicks forward and back
Skate kick
Hopscotch
Knee-high jog with scull
Knee-high jog with hand flutters
Knee-high jog with paddlewheel and reverse
Straddle jog with forearm press, travel back-
   ward and forward
Sprint, travel in a scatter pattern
Knee-high jog, travel in a scatter pattern
Knees to chest with reverse breaststroke and
   breaststroke, travel backward and forward

COOL-DOWN

Crunch with legs in a diamond position
Hip curl with legs in a diamond position
Seated leg lift, hold for 15 seconds
Side-to-side extension with legs in a diamond
   position
Rolling like a ball (Pilates)
Stretch: upper back, pectorals, latissimus dorsi,
   triceps, shoulders, hamstrings

▶ **Deep-Water Lesson Plan 26**

INTERVALS WITH KNEE-HIGH JOG

CLASS OBJECTIVE

Cardiorespiratory fitness

EQUIPMENT

Flotation belt

TEACHING TIP

There are many ways to do intervals. One way is to use a single exercise such as knee-high jog and use different ways of increasing intensity in each set of block choreography.

WARM-UP

Instructor's choice

CONDITIONING PHASE

(A set)

Knee-high jog with shoulder blade squeeze

Knee-high jog with reverse breaststroke and breaststroke, travel backward and forward

Cross-country ski, travel backward and forward

Jumping jacks, clap hands, travel backward and forward

Mini jacks

Jacks tuck

Cossack kick

Interval high-intensity phase: knee-high jog, faster

Interval active recovery phase: knee-high jog

(B set)

Knee-high jog with arm lift to sides

Knee-high jog with double-arm lift and double-arm press-down, travel backward and forward

Cross-country ski with unison sidestroke, travel sideways

Jumping jacks, travel sideways

Jacks cross

Jacks tuck

Frog kick

Interval high-intensity phase: cross-country ski, full ROM

Interval active recovery phase: knee-high jog

(C set)

Knee-high jog with arm curl, palms face direction of motion

Knee-high jog, push forward and crawl stroke, travel backward and forward

Cross-country ski, travel backward and forward

Jumping jacks, clap hands, travel backward and forward

Mini cross

Jacks tuck

Log jump, side to side

Interval high-intensity phase: knee-high jog with elevation

Interval active recovery phase: knee-high jog

(D set)

Knee-high jog with unison jog press

Knee-high jog with forearm press, travel backward and forward

Cross-country ski, diagonal, travel sideways

Jumping jacks, no hands, travel sideways

Seated jacks, 45 degrees

Jacks tuck

Breaststroke kick

Interval high-intensity phase: steep climb

Interval active recovery phase: knee-high jog

COOL-DOWN

Log jump, forward and back

Abdominal pike and spine extension

Abdominal pike and spine extension with legs in a diamond position

Hip curl with legs in a diamond position

Seated jacks, travel backward and forward

Spine twist (Pilates)

Stretch: gastrocnemius, hip flexors, quadriceps, hamstrings, shoulders, neck

▶ Deep-Water Lesson Plan 27

INTERVALS WITH BICYCLE

CLASS OBJECTIVE

Cardiorespiratory fitness

EQUIPMENT

Flotation belt

TEACHING TIP

Participants sweat during water aerobics but may not realize it because of the cooling effect of the water. Encourage them to drink water. For the arm medley, choose any upper-body moves you like.

WARM-UP

Instructor's choice

CONDITIONING PHASE

(A set)

Run tires, reach to the sides

Cross-country ski, travel backward and forward

Cross-country ski

Jumping jacks

Interval high-intensity phase: bicycle, faster

Interval active recovery phase: bicycle, tandem

Flutter kick with scull

Abdominal pike and spine extension

Knee-high jog, palms touch in back

Straddle jog with shoulder blade squeeze

(B set)

Run tires, no hands, travel sideways

Jumping jacks, clap hands, travel backward and forward

Jacks cross

Cross-country ski, corner to corner

Interval high-intensity phase: bicycle, large circles

Interval active recovery phase: bicycle

Flutter kick with sidestroke, travel sideways

Abdominal pike and spine extension, legs wide in front and together in back

Crossover knees

Cossack kick

(C set)

Run tires with alternating paddle pull, travel backward and forward

Cross-country ski, diagonal, travel sideways

Tuck ski

Mini cross

Interval high-intensity phase: bicycle with elevation

Interval active recovery phase: bicycle, tandem

Seated flutter kick with reverse breaststroke and breaststroke, travel backward and forward

Abdominal pike and spine extension, legs together in front and wide in back

Jump rope

Frog kick

(D set)

Knee-high jog with arm medley

(E set)

Seated leg press with unison paddle pull, travel backward and forward

Jumping jacks, travel sideways

Tuck ski, corner to corner

Interval high-intensity phase: bicycle, climb a hill

Interval active recovery phase: bicycle

COOL-DOWN

Flutter kick up to L position and down to upright

Abdominal pike and spine extension, legs wide in front and wide in back with tuck in center

Hip curl with alternating knees

Crunch with legs in a diamond position

Jumping jacks, side-lying

Bicycle, side-lying, in a circle and reverse

Stretch: hip flexors, quadriceps, hamstrings, upper back, pectorals, shoulders

▶ Deep-Water Lesson Plan 28

INTERVALS WITH CROSS-COUNTRY SKI

CLASS OBJECTIVE

Cardiorespiratory fitness

EQUIPMENT

Flotation belt

TEACHING TIP

Cross-country ski works well with all of the ways to increase intensity, which makes it a good exercise to use in interval training. For the arm medley, choose any upper-body moves you like.

WARM-UP

Instructor's choice

CONDITIONING PHASE

(A set)

Knee-high jog with jog press

Straddle jog with jog press in front

Run tires, reach to the sides

Jumping jacks

Cross-country ski and jumping jacks, alternate

Interval high-intensity phase: mini ski, faster

Interval active recovery phase: cross-country ski

Cossack kick

(B set)

Knee-high jog, scull in front and scull arms down, travel backward and forward

Straddle jog with reverse breaststroke and breaststroke, travel backward and forward

Run tires with alternating paddle pull, travel backward and forward

Jumping jacks, clap hands, travel backward and forward

Cross-country ski and jumping jacks, alternate

Interval high-intensity phase: cross-country ski, full ROM

Interval active recovery phase: cross-country ski

Cossack kick

(C set)

Knee-high jog with arm medley

(D set)

Knee-high jog, diagonal, travel sideways

Straddle jog with single-arm sweep, travel sideways

Over the barrel, travel sideways

Jumping jacks, travel sideways

Cross-country ski and jumping jacks, alternate

Interval high-intensity phase: cross-country ski with elevation

Interval active recovery phase: cross-country ski

Cossack kick

(E set)

Crossover knees

Cossack kick with alternating legs

In in, out out

Jumping jacks upright, then 45 degrees, then seated, then 45 degrees, then upright

Cross-country ski and jumping jacks, alternate

Interval high-intensity phase: cross-country ski with power

Interval active recovery phase: cross-country ski

Cossack kick

COOL-DOWN

Knee-high jog, side-lying, travel

Frog kick

Seated leg press with unison paddle pull, travel backward and forward

Seated jacks, travel backward and forward

L position with reverse breaststroke and breaststroke, travel backward and forward

Seated reverse breaststroke and breaststroke, travel backward and forward

Dolphin, travel backward; rock climb, travel forward

Stretch: hip flexors, gastrocnemius, hamstrings, outer thigh, lower back, shoulders

▶ Deep-Water Lesson Plan 29

INTERVALS WITH SPEED

CLASS OBJECTIVE

Cardiorespiratory fitness

EQUIPMENT

Flotation belt

TEACHING TIP

There are many ways to do intervals. One option is to apply one way of increasing intensity to different exercises in each set of block choreography. If you increase intensity with speed, encourage your participants not to lose their range of motion and make the move smaller. For the arm medley, choose any upper-body moves you like.

WARM-UP

Instructor's choice

CONDITIONING PHASE

(A set)

Bicycle, scull in front and scull arms down, travel backward and forward

Flutter kick up to L position and down to upright

Seated reverse breaststroke and breaststroke, travel backward and forward

High kick

Ankle touch, feet wide apart

Hopscotch, feet wide apart

Knee-high jog with unison push forward and standing row, travel backward and forward

Crossover knees

Interval high-intensity phase: knee-high jog, faster

Interval active recovery phase: knee-high jog

(B set)

Bicycle with sidestroke, travel sideways

Flutter kick up to L position and down to upright

Seated reverse breaststroke and breaststroke, travel backward and forward

High kick

Ankle touch, feet close together

Hopscotch, feet close together

Cross-country ski, travel backward and forward

Mini ski

Interval high-intensity phase: cross-country ski, faster

Interval active recovery phase: cross-country ski

(C set)

Knee-high jog with arm medley

(D set)

Bicycle with reverse breaststroke and breaststroke, travel backward and forward

Flutter kick up to L position and down to upright

Seated reverse breaststroke and breaststroke, travel backward and forward

High kick

Ankle touch and hopscotch, alternate

Jumping jacks, clap hands, travel backward and forward

Mini jacks

Interval high-intensity phase: jumping jacks, faster

Interval active recovery phase: jumping jacks

(E set)

Bicycle, diagonal, travel sideways

Flutter kick up to L position and down to upright

Seated reverse breaststroke and breaststroke, travel backward and forward

High kick

Ankle touch, one ankle only and hopscotch, one heel only; alternate

Bicycle with forearm press, travel backward and forward

Bicycle, small circles

Interval high-intensity phase: bicycle, faster

Interval active recovery phase: bicycle

COOL-DOWN

Pelvic tilt, upright

Log jump, side to side

Log jump, one side

Side crunch from a kneeling position

V-sit

The hundred (Pilates)

Stretch: hamstrings, outer thigh, inner thigh, quadriceps, latissimus dorsi, shoulders

▶ Deep-Water Lesson Plan 30

INTERVALS WITH ROM

CLASS OBJECTIVE

Cardiorespiratory fitness

EQUIPMENT

Flotation belt

TEACHING TIP

When you increase intensity by increasing range of motion, encourage participants to go to their personal full range of motion, even if theirs is different from those of others in the class. For the arm medley, choose any upper-body moves you like.

WARM-UP

Instructor's choice

CONDITIONING PHASE

(A set)

Straddle jog

Diamonds, upright

Run tires, no hands, travel sideways

Sprint

Kick forward with reverse breaststroke and breaststroke, travel backward and forward

Kick forward with crossovers

Kick forward, doubles

Interval high-intensity phase: high kick

Interval active recovery phase: kick forward

(B set)

Straddle jog

Cossack kick

Run tires with sidestroke, travel sideways

Sprint

Jumping jacks, travel sideways

Jumping jacks, palms touch in front and in back

Jacks tuck

Interval high-intensity phase: jacks cross, full ROM

Interval active recovery phase: jumping jacks

(C set)

Straddle jog

Cossack kick with alternating legs

Run tires with paddle pull, travel backward and forward

Sprint

Cross-country ski, travel backward and forward

Cross-country ski with forearm press, side to side

Tuck ski, corner to corner

Interval high-intensity phase: cross-country ski, full ROM

Interval active recovery phase: cross-country ski

(D set)

Knee-high jog with arm medley

COOL-DOWN

Straddle jog

Diamonds, upright and seated, alternate

Seated leg press, travel backward

Bicycle, no hands, travel forward

Seated jacks, travel backward and forward

Seated jacks, open and close doors

Seated triple crossover

Seated jacks cross, full ROM

Hip curl, L position

Crunch, V position

Side-to-side extension, R leg only

Side-to-side extension, L leg only

Stretch: gastrocnemius, hip flexors, quadriceps, hamstrings, inner thigh, shoulders

► Deep-Water Lesson Plan 31

INTERVALS WITH ELEVATION

CLASS OBJECTIVES

Cardiorespiratory fitness and muscular strength and endurance

EQUIPMENT

Flotation belt and dumbbells (optional)

TEACHING TIP

When you are demonstrating one-sided moves on the deck, participants will be able to follow you better if you use the mirror image technique. Tell them to use the right leg, but demonstrate with your left leg. If dumbbells are unavailable for the strength training section at the beginning of the cool-down, ask participants to push hard against the water while jogging for stability.

WARM-UP

Knee-high jog with jog press

Knee-high jog with unison jog press

Tuck ski

Cross-country ski, knees bent 90 degrees

Cross-country ski

Bicycle with standing row

Bicycle with crossovers

Straddle jog with paddlewheel

Straddle jog with scull

CONDITIONING PHASE

(A set)

Skate kick

Ankle touch

High kick

One leg kicks forward and back

Knee-high jog with shoulder blade squeeze

Knee-high jog, palms touch in back

Knee-high jog with triceps extension

Knee-high jog, one knee only

Knee-high jog, diagonal, travel sideways

Interval high-intensity phase: knee-high jog with elevation

Interval active recovery phase: knee-high jog

Knee-high jog, side-lying, travel

(B set)

Skate kick

Ankle touch

High kick

One leg kicks forward and back

Cross-country ski, clap hands

Cross-country ski with lat pull-down

Cross-country ski with alternating arm curl

Tuck ski

Cross-country ski, diagonal, travel sideways

Interval high-intensity phase: cross-country ski with elevation

Interval active recovery phase: cross-country ski

Cross-country ski, side-lying, travel

(C set)

Skate kick

Ankle touch

High kick

One leg kicks forward and back

Bicycle with shoulder blade squeeze

Bicycle, palms touch in back

Bicycle with triceps extension

Bicycle, one leg only

Bicycle, diagonal, travel sideways

Interval high-intensity phase: bicycle with elevation

Interval active recovery phase: bicycle

Bicycle, side-lying, travel

(D set)

Skate kick

Ankle touch

High kick

One leg kicks forward and back

Straddle jog, clap hands

Straddle jog, palms touch in front

Straddle jog with arm curl

Frog kick

Straddle jog, diagonal, travel sideways

Interval high-intensity phase: straddle jog with elevation

Interval active recovery phase: straddle jog

Seated leg press with unison paddle pull, travel backward and forward

COOL-DOWN

(With dumbbells)

Knee-high jog with shoulder blade squeeze, dumbbells upright

Knee-high jog, dumbbells touch in back

Knee-high jog with triceps extension

Side-to-side extension, dumbbells extended to sides

Abdominal pike and spine extension, dumbbells together in front on the surface of the water

Stretch: shoulders, upper back, latissimus dorsi, triceps, hip flexors, hamstrings

▶ Deep-Water Lesson Plan 32

INTERVALS WITH POWER

CLASS OBJECTIVE

Cardiorespiratory fitness

EQUIPMENT

Flotation belt

TEACHING TIP

It is sometimes difficult to teach adding power to a move. Use as many power words as you can think of, such as *force, effort, energy, intensity, make waves, might, use your muscles, push hard, strength, vigor,* and *high voltage.* It may also help to get in the water with your class and demonstrate.

WARM-UP

Jumping jacks

Jacks tuck

Tuck ski

Cross-country ski

Cross-country ski, knees bent 90 degrees

Bicycle with scull

Heel jog with scull

Knee-high jog with jog press

Knee-high jog with reverse breaststroke and breaststroke, travel backward and forward

Seated reverse breaststroke and breaststroke, travel backward and forward

CONDITIONING PHASE

(A set)

Jumping jacks, travel sideways

Jacks cross

One leg kicks side

Interval high-intensity phase: jumping jacks with power

Interval active recovery phase: jumping jacks

Knee-high jog with reverse breaststroke with power and breaststroke, travel backward and forward

Seated reverse breaststroke and breaststroke, travel backward and forward

(B set)

Cross-country ski, travel backward and forward

Cross-country ski, corner to corner

One leg kicks forward and back

Interval high-intensity phase: cross-country ski with power

Interval active recovery phase: cross-country ski

Knee-high jog with reverse breaststroke and breaststroke with power, travel backward and forward

Seated reverse breaststroke and breaststroke, travel backward and forward

(C set)

Bicycle with unison arm swing, travel backward and forward

Bicycle, tandem

Bicycle, one leg only

Interval high-intensity phase: bicycle, climb a hill

Interval active recovery phase: bicycle

Knee-high jog with reverse breaststroke with power and breaststroke with power, travel backward and forward

Seated reverse breaststroke and breaststroke, travel backward and forward

(D set)

Knee-high jog with double-arm lift and double-arm press-down with power, travel backward and forward

Ankle touch

Knee-high jog, one knee only, with sidestroke, travel sideways

Interval high-intensity phase: steep climb

Interval active recovery phase: knee-high jog

Knee-high jog with reverse breaststroke and breaststroke, travel backward and forward

Seated reverse breaststroke with power and breaststroke with power, travel backward and forward

(E set)

Heel jog with forearm press, travel backward and forward

Hopscotch

Mermaid

Interval high-intensity phase: seated kick with power, travel forward

Interval active recovery phase: seated kick

COOL-DOWN

Knee-high jog with reverse breaststroke and breaststroke, travel backward and forward

Seated reverse breaststroke and breaststroke, travel backward and forward

Log jump, forward and back

Log jump, side to side

Log jump, side to side, doubles

One leg—knee lift, kick forward, side knee lift, kick side, heel lift, kick back

Stretch: hip flexors, quadriceps, hamstrings, outer thigh, upper back, pectorals

▶ **Deep-Water Lesson Plan 33**

INTERVALS WITH SPEED AND ELEVATION

CLASS OBJECTIVE

Cardiorespiratory fitness

EQUIPMENT

Flotation belt

TEACHING TIP

To add variety and challenge to your interval training, experiment with different ways of increasing intensity, using several different exercises. This lesson plan uses speed and elevation to increase intensity with knee-high jog, flutter kick, cross-country ski and run tires.

Limit the length of time your participants work with the hands overhead to 15 to 30 seconds, or cue raising the hands to just above the ears. Participants with high blood pressure should not raise their hands above their heads.

WARM-UP

Instructor's choice

CONDITIONING PHASE

(A set)

Kick forward

Jumping jacks

Heel jog

Skate kick

Knee-high jog, scull in front and scull arms down, travel backward and forward

Interval high-intensity phase: knee-high jog, faster

Interval active recovery phase: knee-high jog

Interval high-intensity phase: knee-high jog with elevation

Interval active recovery phase: knee-high jog

Interval high-intensity phase: knee-high jog, faster, hands up

Interval active recovery phase: knee-high jog

Knee-high jog with breaststroke 4× and reverse breaststroke 4×, alternate

Knee-high jog with breaststroke and reverse breaststroke, alternate

(B set)

High kick, travel backward

Jumping jacks, clap hands, travel forward and backward

Heel jog with crawl stroke and push forward, travel forward and backward

Skate kick, hands behind back, travel forward

Flutter kick with unison sidestroke, travel sideways

Interval high-intensity phase: flutter kick, faster

Interval active recovery phase: flutter kick

Interval high-intensity phase: flutter kick with elevation

Interval active recovery phase: flutter kick

Interval high-intensity phase: flutter kick, faster, hands up

Interval active recovery phase: flutter kick

Knee-high jog with lat pull-down

Knee-high jog with double-arm press-down

Knee-high jog with lat pull-down and double-arm press-down, alternate

(C set)

Mermaid

Jacks tuck

Breaststroke kick

Tuck ski together

Cross-country ski, travel backward and forward

Interval high-intensity phase: mini ski, faster

Interval active recovery phase: cross-country ski

Interval high-intensity phase: cross-country ski with elevation

Interval active recovery phase: cross-country ski

Interval high-intensity phase: cross-country ski, faster

Interval active recovery phase: cross-country ski

Knee-high jog with arm curl

Knee-high jog with triceps extension

Knee-high jog with arm curl, palms face direction of motion

(D set)

Seated kick, travel backward

Seated jacks, travel forward and backward

Seated kick, travel forward

Tuck ski together, side-lying, travel

Over the barrel, travel sideways

Interval high-intensity phase: run tires, faster

Interval active recovery phase: run tires

Interval high-intensity phase: run tires with elevation

Interval active recovery phase: run tires

Interval high-intensity phase: run tires, faster, hands up

Interval active recovery phase: run tires

Knee-high jog with forearm press

Knee-high jog with forearm press, side to side

COOL-DOWN

Seated jacks

Seated mini cross

Seated triple crossover

Crunch, V position

Eight short crunches and two long crunches

Stretch: hamstrings, quadriceps, hip flexors, pectorals, latissimus dorsi, triceps, shoulders

▶ Deep-Water Lesson Plan 34

INTERVALS WITH ELEVATION AND POWER

CLASS OBJECTIVE

Cardiorespiratory fitness

EQUIPMENT

Flotation belt

TEACHING TIP

Just for fun, try having your participants move quickly from one working position to another. They can alternate flutter kick and flutter kick with elevation. They can flutter kick side-lying and then roll over to the other side to continue the side-lying flutter kick. They can flutter kick in an L position, then bend the knees and go into a seated kick, and then straighten the body and flutter kick upright lifting the shoulders out of the water.

WARM-UP

Instructor's choice

CONDITIONING PHASE

(A set)

Seated kick, palms touch in back

Seated flutter kick

Flutter down to upright

Crossover knees

Ankle touch

Straddle jog with crossovers

Straddle jog, clap hands, travel backward

Sprint, travel in a zigzag

Cross-country ski, travel backward and forward

Interval high-intensity phase: cross-country ski with elevation

Interval active recovery phase: cross-country ski

Interval high-intensity phase: knee-high jog with elevation

Interval active recovery phase: knee-high jog

Flutter kick and flutter kick with elevation, alternate

Cross-country ski, side-lying, travel

(B set)

Seated kick, travel backward and forward

Seated flutter kick, no hands and with unison arm swing, travel backward and forward

Flutter down to upright

Crossover knees

Ankle touch, doubles

Straddle jog with double-arm press-down

Knee-high jog with unison arm swing, travel backward

Sprint, travel in a zigzag

Cross-country ski, diagonal, travel sideways

Interval high-intensity phase: cross-country ski with power

Interval active recovery phase: cross-country ski

Interval high-intensity phase: steep climb

Interval active recovery phase: knee-high jog

Flutter kick, side-lying R, roll over and flutter kick, side-lying L, travel

Knee-high jog, side-lying, travel

(C set)

Seated kick, one leg only

Seated flutter kick, one leg only

Flutter down to upright

Crossover knees

Ankle touch R

Straddle jog, open and close doors

Straddle jog with reverse breaststroke, travel backward

Sprint, travel in a zigzag

Cross-country ski, travel backward and forward

Interval high-intensity phase: cross-country ski with elevation

Interval active recovery phase: cross-country ski

Interval high-intensity phase: knee-high jog with elevation

Interval active recovery phase: knee-high jog

Seated flutter kick, seated kick, and flutter kick with elevation; alternate

Tuck ski together, side-lying, travel

(D set)

Mermaid with scull

Flutter kick up to L position and down to upright 4×

Crossover knees

Ankle touch L

Straddle jog with forearm press

Knee-high jog, push forward, travel backward

Sprint, travel in a zigzag

Cross-country ski, diagonal, travel sideways

Interval high-intensity phase: cross-country ski with power

Interval active recovery phase: cross-country ski

Interval high-intensity phase: steep climb

Interval active recovery phase: knee-high jog

COOL-DOWN

Flutter kick, side-lying, travel

Bicycle, side-lying, travel

Abdominal pike and spine extension

Abdominal pike and spine extension with legs in a diamond position

Side-to-side extension with legs in a diamond position

Hip curl from a kneeling position

Stretch: gastrocnemius, hip flexors, quadriceps, hamstrings, shoulders, pectorals

▶ Deep-Water Lesson Plan 35

INTERVALS WITH SPEED, ROM, AND ELEVATION

CLASS OBJECTIVE

Cardiorespiratory fitness

EQUIPMENT

Flotation belt

TEACHING TIP

Try organizing two exercises in a pyramid, as follows: a 8×, b 8×, a 4×, b 4×, a 2×, b 2×, a, b. You can also reverse the order, beginning with "a" and "b" alternating and working up to eight times. For the arm medley, choose any upper-body moves you like.

WARM-UP

Knee-high jog with jog press

Knee-high jog, palms touch in back

Straddle jog with shoulder blade squeeze

Heel jog with triceps extension

Knee-high jog with scull

Knee-high jog, scull in front and scull arms down, travel backward and forward

Knee-high jog with side arm curl, travel sideways

CONDITIONING PHASE

(A set)

Flutter kick

Kick forward, push forward and crawl stroke, travel backward and forward

Cossack kick with sidestroke, travel sideways

Flutter kick, side-lying, travel

Kick to the corners

Kick forward and kick to the corners, pyramid (see explanation of this term in the teaching tip for this lesson plan)

Interval high-intensity phase: flutter kick, faster

Interval active recovery phase: flutter kick

Interval high-intensity phase: high kick

Interval active recovery phase: flutter kick, feet pointed and flexed, alternate

Interval high-intensity phase: flutter kick with elevation

Interval active recovery phase: flutter kick up to L position and down to upright

Flutter kick

(B set)

Cross-country ski

Jumping jacks, clap hands, travel backward and forward

Straddle jog with single-arm sweep, travel sideways

Cross-country ski, side-lying, travel

Jumping jacks

Cross-country ski and jumping jacks, pyramid

Interval high-intensity phase: cross-country ski, faster

Interval active recovery phase: cross-country ski

Interval high-intensity phase: cross-country ski, full ROM

Interval active recovery phase: tuck ski

Interval high-intensity phase: cross-country ski with elevation

Interval active recovery phase: tuck ski, corner to corner

Cross-country ski

(C set)

Knee-high jog with arm medley

(D set)

Bicycle

Run tires with paddle pull, travel backward and forward

Over the barrel, travel sideways

Bicycle, side-lying, travel

Run tires

Knee-high jog and run tires, pyramid

Interval high-intensity phase: bicycle, faster

Interval active recovery phase: bicycle

Interval high-intensity phase: bicycle, large circles

Interval active recovery phase: bicycle, one leg only

Interval high-intensity phase: bicycle with elevation

Interval active recovery phase: bicycle, tandem

COOL-DOWN

Bicycle

Side-to-side extension

Abdominal pike and spine extension

Extension forward, R, back, L, and reverse

Stretch: inner thigh, outer thigh, hamstrings, quadriceps, obliques, shoulders, triceps

▶ Deep-Water Lesson Plan 36

INTERVALS WITH SPEED, ROM, ELEVATION, AND POWER

CLASS OBJECTIVE

Cardiorespiratory fitness

EQUIPMENT

Flotation belt

TEACHING TIP

Sometimes participants are more likely to drink water if you offer them water breaks. Don't forget to drink water yourself!

WARM-UP

Knee-high jog with jog press

Seated kick with scull

Knee-high jog with scull

Knee-high jog, scull in front and scull arms down, travel backward and forward 2×

Knee-high jog with side arm curl, travel sideways

CONDITIONING PHASE

(A set)

One leg kicks forward and back

Ankle touch

Hopscotch

Heel jog with shoulder blade squeeze

Cross-country ski, corner to corner

Jumping jacks, clap hands

Knee-high jog with reverse breaststroke and breaststroke, travel backward and forward

Interval high-intensity phase: knee-high jog, faster

Interval active recovery phase: knee-high jog

Interval high-intensity phase: mini ski, faster

Interval active recovery phase: knee-high jog

Interval high-intensity phase: knee-high jog, faster, hands up

Interval active recovery phase: knee-high jog

(B set)

One leg kicks forward and back

Ankle touch, one ankle only

Hopscotch, one heel only

Heel jog with shoulder blade squeeze

Cross-country ski with windshield wiper arms

Jumping jacks, palms touch in front

Knee-high jog with unison arm swing, travel backward and forward

Interval high-intensity phase: high kick

Interval active recovery phase: kick forward

Interval high-intensity phase: cross-country ski, full ROM

Interval active recovery phase: kick forward

Interval high-intensity phase: high kick 7×, tuck and turn

Interval active recovery phase: kick forward

(C set)

One leg kicks forward and back

Ankle touch, doubles

Hopscotch, doubles

Heel jog with shoulder blade squeeze

Cross-country ski with alternating arm curl

Jumping jacks, open and close doors

Knee-high jog, push forward and triceps pressback, travel backward and forward

Interval high-intensity phase: bicycle with elevation

Interval active recovery phase: bicycle

Interval high-intensity phase: cross-country ski with elevation

Interval active recovery phase: bicycle

Interval high-intensity phase: bicycle with elevation, travel in a circle

Interval active recovery phase: bicycle

(D set)

One leg kicks forward and back

Ankle touch, one ankle only and hopscotch, one heel only; alternate

Heel jog with shoulder blade squeeze

Cross-country ski with forearm press, side to side

Jumping jacks, palms touch in back

Knee-high jog with forearm press, travel backward and forward

Interval high-intensity phase: steep climb

Interval active recovery phase: knee-high jog

Interval high-intensity phase: cross-country ski with power

Interval active recovery phase: knee-high jog

Interval high-intensity phase: steep climb 4× with quarter turn

Interval active recovery phase: knee-high jog

COOL-DOWN

Knee-high jog with scull

Knee-high jog, scull in front and scull arms down, travel backward and forward

Knee-high jog, diagonal, travel sideways

Side-to-side extension

Bicycle, side-lying, in a circle

Hip curl, V position

Crunch, V position

V-sit

Stretch: pectorals, upper back, shoulders, hip flexors, hamstrings, quadriceps, outer thigh

REFERENCE

YMCA. (2000). *YMCA Water Fitness for Health.* Champaign, IL: Human Kinetics.

GLOSSARY

abduction—Movement of a joint away from the midline of the body.

active recovery phase—A short break during interval training in which the intensity is decreased.

add-on choreography—A type of choreography in which participants perform a set of exercises, add on a new set, and then repeat all the sets from the beginning.

adduction—Movement of a joint toward the midline of the body.

audible cue—A spoken instruction, hand clap, or whistle.

block choreography—A type of choreography in which the pattern set up in the first set is repeated with variations in each succeeding set.

Borg's scale of perceived exertion—A method of measuring intensity during exercise by rating how hard the person is working on a scale of 6 to 20 or 1 to 10.

cardiorespiratory fitness—The ability of the heart and lungs to deliver oxygen to the working muscles.

center of buoyancy—The center of the volume of a body in water, usually located in the chest.

center of gravity—The center of the body's mass, usually located in the pelvic area.

choreography—A way to organize exercises in a water fitness class to give them logic and flow and make them easy to remember.

circuit class—A type of strength training class in which work stations are set up around the edge of the pool.

class objective—The goal for participants to accomplish during a water fitness class.

conditioning phase—The main section of a water fitness class.

continuous training—Training that brings participants up to their target heart rates and keeps them there for the duration of the conditioning phase.

cool-down—The last part of a water fitness class in which participants slowly recover from the work they have done in the conditioning phase.

core strength—The strength of the trunk muscles, which maintain posture.

cue—A signal used to let participants know what exercise to perform.

dynamic stretch—A stretch performed by moving the muscles slowly through their full range of motion.

elevation—A way to increase intensity in deep water by using a scull to lift the shoulders out of the water while working the legs very hard, or by pulling the arms and legs together forcefully enough to lift the shoulders out of the water.

flotation device—A deep-water belt, cuffs for the upper arms, or cuffs for the ankles.

hands up—Raising the arms out of the water in deep water to make the body sink and force the legs to work harder.

heart rate chart—A chart that estimates target heart rates based on population averages.

high-intensity phase—The part of interval training in which intensity is increased to bring the heart rate into the upper level of the target heart rate.

interval training—Increasing intensity so that the heart rate climbs into the upper level of the target heart rate for a short time before decreasing the intensity to let the heart rate go back into the mid- or lower level.

linear choreography—A type of choreography in which the exercises have no repetition or very little repetition.

long-lever move—Using a straight limb to increase the resistance in water.

maximum heart rate—The highest your heart rate can go; determined by using the formula 220 minus age.

modified circuit class—A type of circuit class in which rhythmic exercises are alternated with strength training exercises.

muscular endurance—The ability of a muscle to exert force repeatedly.

muscular strength—The amount of force a muscle can exert.

neutral position—A position in shallow water in which the hips and knees are flexed and the shoulders are at the surface of the water.

overload—Placing a greater demand on the muscles than normal to increase strength.

physical cue—Pointing to the muscle participants should focus on.

power—A way to increase intensity by pushing harder against the resistance of the water.

pressor response—The tendency of the heart to work harder to pump blood against gravity when the arms are raised overhead.

range of motion (ROM)—The distance and direction that a joint can move to its full potential. The intensity of water exercises can be increased by using long levers (arms and legs slightly flexed) through their full range of motion.

rebounding—Jumping.

ROM—See *range of motion (ROM)*.

scull—A stabilizing move in water in which the hands sweep outward with the thumbs angled down and inward with the thumbs angled up.

short-lever move—Using a bent limb to decrease the resistance in water.

speed—The velocity at which movement is performed. The intensity of water exercises can be increased by increasing velocity without compromising range of motion.

static stretch—A muscle stretch that is held for 10 to 30 seconds.

suspended moves—Moves performed without touching the bottom of the pool; a way to increase exercise intensity in shallow water.

talk test—A method of measuring intensity during exercise by checking whether one is breathing too hard to be able to talk.

target heart rate—The heart rate at which participants should work during exercise; between 60 and 80 percent of maximum heart rate.

travel—Moving through the water from one part of the pool to another.

variations on a theme—A type of linear choreography in which two or three exercises are worked through multiple variations.

visual cue—A physical demonstration or hand signal.

warm-up—The first part of a water fitness class in which participants adjust their body temperatures to the water temperature, warm up their muscles, and increase their heart rates in preparation for the workout.

water tempo—The appropriate rate of speed in water.

ABOUT THE AUTHOR

Christine Alexander is a water fitness instructor for the City of Plano Parks and Recreation Department at Oak Point Recreation Center. She teaches additional classes for the City of Addison, the City of McKinney, and the YMCA. She is a nationally certified water fitness instructor and an instructor-trainer through the United States Water Fitness Association. She is also a certified water fitness instructor through the YMCA of the USA and an Arthritis Foundation Aquatic Program instructor. She has served as a board member for the Metroplex Association of Aquatic Professionals, including a three-year term as president of that organization. As an advocate for water fitness, Alexander regularly presents master workouts and has conducted her own introductory course for water fitness instructors. She also enjoys mentoring beginning water fitness instructors.

Alexander lives in Plano, Texas, with her husband, Jim. In her free time, she enjoys weight training, cooking healthy meals, and organic gardening.

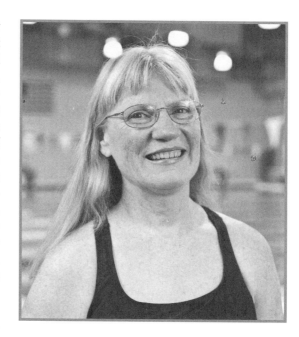

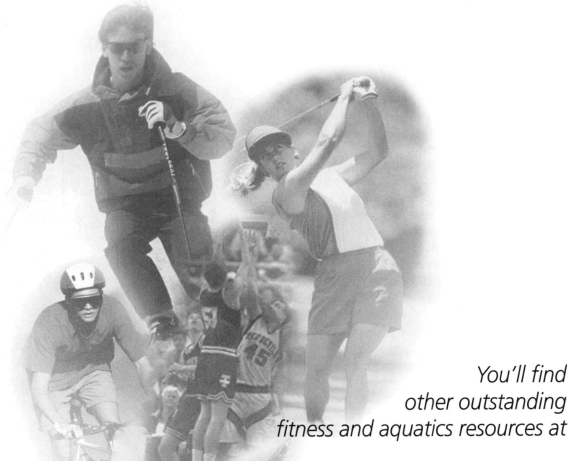